YOGA
DECONSTRUCTED®

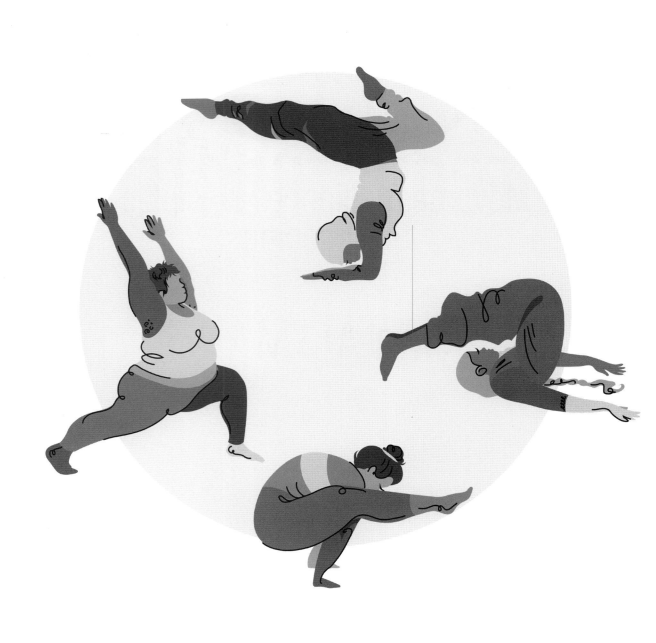

YOGA
DECONSTRUCTED®
Movement science principles for teaching

Trina ALTMAN

Forewords
Jules Mitchell
Carrie Owerko

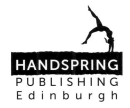

HANDSPRING
PUBLISHING
Edinburgh

HANDSPRING PUBLISHING LIMITED
The Old Manse, Fountainhall,
Pencaitland, East Lothian
EH34 5EY, United Kingdom
Tel: +44 1875 341 859
Website: www.handspringpublishing.com

First published 2021 in the United Kingdom by Handspring Publishing

ISBN 978-1-912085-44-6
ISBN (Kindle ebook) 978-1-912085-45-3

British Library Cataloguing in Publication Data
A catalogue record for this book is available from the British Library

Library of Congress Cataloguing in Publication Data
A catalog record for this book is available from the Library of Congress

Notice
Neither the Publisher nor the Author assume any responsibility for any loss or injury and/or damage to persons or property arising out of or relating to any use of the material contained in this book. It is the responsibility of the treating practitioner, relying on independent expertise and knowledge of the patient, to determine the best treatment and method of application for the patient.

All reasonable efforts have been made to obtain copyright clearance for illustrations in the book for which the authors or publishers do not own the rights. If you believe that one of your illustrations has been used without such clearance please contact the publishers and we will ensure that appropriate credit is given in the next reprint.

Commissioning Editor Sarena Wolfaard
Project Manager Morven Dean
Copy-editor Susan Stuart
Design Bruce Hogarth
Cover art and illustrations Dionna Gary Bunn - www.designedbydg.net
Indexer Aptara, India
Typesetter DSM, India
Printer Melita, Malta

The
Publisher's
policy is to use
paper manufactured
from sustainable forests

CONTENTS

ABOUT THE AUTHOR

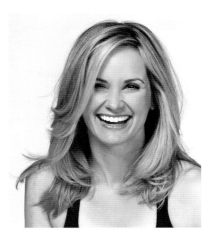

TRINA ALTMAN, BA, E-RYT 500, YACEP, NCPT, STOTT PILATES® certified instructor, is the creator of Yoga Deconstructed® and Pilates Deconstructed®, which shows movement teachers and clinicians how to modernize their teaching and create a more sustainable practice through an interdisciplinary approach based on current movement science.

Trina has over a decade of teaching experience and has taught throughout North America, Central America, Europe, and Australia.

Trina has presented at Kripalu, PURE YOGA® NYC, Yogaworks, SYTAR, the Yoga Alliance Leadership Conference, ECA, Momentum Fest and multiple yoga conferences. She also created and taught a Pilates continuing education course for physical therapists and was part of the faculty for the Brain Longevity® conference at UCLA. Her work has been published in Yoga Journal, Yoga International, and Pilates Style magazine and her classes and courses have been featured on Yoga International, Yoga Anytime and Fusion Pilates EDU.

She also consulted for Equinox to help develop their signature program Best Stretch Ever, which utilizes the mobility stick to improve functional range of motion, body awareness, and total body strength. Her teaching fosters body cognition and self-discovery, firmly grounded in anatomical awareness.

For more information on Trina and her online classes and courses, visit trinaaltman.com

FOREWORD *by Jules Mitchell*

Trina Altman sets the proverbial record straight when it comes to the art of designing classes. Her kindhearted approach invites you into an intricate unraveling of the unvalidated status quo. She speaks to the reader as a friend and comrade, sharing her own struggles along her teaching journey when her continued education did not align with the rules that had been laid out for her. This book does not tell you *what* to do, instead it tells you *how* to do what you want with purpose. And that, in itself, is a huge accomplishment.

I first met Trina close to ten years ago when we were both at a major turning point of our teaching paths. We had both found our own individual mentors that we truly admired, who had shown us there was another way, yet we both had our own ideas about our futures. I was organizing an event and remember inviting Trina to teach a few workshops. She was confident, and incredibly clear, about the content she was offering and her expectations for the event parameters. That assertiveness, combined with an enormous commitment to those lucky enough to study under her, is what fills the pages that lie ahead. *Yoga Deconstructed*® is brimming with information on what it can look like to compassionately teach an embodied practice to wide variety of populations.

My own teaching path has sent me to across the globe, providing continuing education to yoga teachers both online and in person. I often find I share a significant student base with Trina, meaning I am witness to the complexity and progressive nature of this audience. You are curious and sharp-minded. You are open to criticism, both of yourselves and of systems that have failed your communities. You demand change yet respect the roots of the practice. You are keenly aware of the inequalities that are present within the hierarchies of modern postural yoga. On occasion, Trina, herself has been a student in my courses. I learned that she too, shares the qualities of this cohort. She is not teaching from above, but from within.

In *Yoga Deconstructed*®, Trina guides you through her process in a step-by-step manner, pausing frequently to give an abundance of practical examples. You will want to read this book in an environment where you can get on the floor and experience everything she offers! Additionally, she frequently provides teacher considerations, where you have the opportunity to assimilate the content into your own teaching style and educational background before moving on. Trina starts with a foundation, progresses into the more complex topics, then introduces a powerful awareness tool. It all comes together as she walks you through building a sequence from start to finish. Presenting the book in the same way in which she teaches a class is brilliant! It is a must-read for any post-lineage yoga teacher.

Jules Mitchell MS, LMT, RYT
Yoga Educator, Research & Adjunct Faculty
Arizona State University
Author: Yoga Biomechanics:
Stretching Redefined
www.JulesMitchell.com
August 2020

FOREWORD *by Carrie Owerko*

Several years ago, a student I met in a workshop that I was teaching asked me if Trina Altman and I knew each other. She remarked that there were many aspects of our teaching that were similar. Excited to get to know a kindred spirit, I did a little investigating via social media. Soon after, Trina attended a training session that I was teaching in Los Angeles. We spent time in passionate conversation about all things yoga and movement, and became fast friends, united in our embrace of a science-based, yet creative, ever evolving, unconventional approach to yoga practice.

Trina is a gentle rebel. Open-minded and open-hearted, yet willing to dive deep and take a stand for what she believes is important.

Yoga Deconstructed® is a singular example of such a stand. It is an extremely valuable and important contribution, one that is distinct among the plethora of yoga books that are out in the world. Her book fills a vital gap in what is currently available, especially for the person who has been injured and has gone through physical therapy, yet might not feel ready to participate fully in a traditional yoga class.

Trina shares her own history with pain and injury and what she has learned about the value of cross training and gradually increasing one's capacity to withstand the stress of physical activity (versus avoiding the activity – which is often enjoyable – and as a result becoming less capable, resilient, and happy or fulfilled as a person).

Yoga Deconstructed® is empowering rather than fear-mongering or dogmatic. She gives readers easy-to-understand principles and information that can help guide them in their own process of returning to the yoga studio, or their favorite activity, with confidence.

If you are a yoga teacher, this book will give you basic, practical information drawn from exercise science that will help you help your students help themselves: the greatest gift a teacher can impart. If you are a student, especially someone with a history of pain and/or injury, this book will help you become your own teacher, so that even within the context of a group yoga class, you can help yourself to practice in a way that honors where you are on any given day, building trust in your own ability to progress or regress an asana or movement, and honor your unique experience and yoga journey.

Trina has written an intelligent, compassionate, and inspiring book. It is as smart, open-minded and open-hearted as she is, something that the ever-expanding (and hopefully ever-evolving) yoga community could greatly use.

Carrie Owerko BFA, CMA, CYIT, C-IAYT, FRCms
Laban Movement Analyst, Yoga Therapist,
Certified Senior teacher of Iyengar Yoga,
Functional Range Conditioning Mobility Specialist
www.carrieowerko.com
August 2020

PREFACE

My initial introduction to yoga was through a semester-long class at Brown University. It was the first time I'd ever experienced movement in a way that was not competitive or aesthetically driven. At the time, I had no idea that I would one day become a yoga teacher. I simply saw it as a reprieve from the stress of studying and job searching. However, upon reflection, I realize that this class marked an initial shift in the lens through which I viewed and experienced movement. Years later, I took a class with Kirsten Collins in New Haven, Connecticut, and I thought to myself, "One day, I want to do what she is doing." At the time though, I didn't think it was possible. Three years later, I found myself still yearning to teach, but was mired in self-doubt. It was only because Farzad, my now husband, urged me to sign up for a 200-hour teacher training that I found the courage to take the leap.

Some time between completing my teacher training and transitioning into the role of a full-time yoga teacher, I began to experience pain in my body. Sometimes, the pain ran down into my forearm, hand, and wrist. Other times, it centered more in my jaw, neck, upper back, and shoulders. It plagued me throughout the day, even when I wasn't practicing yoga poses. I didn't know it at the time, but I was hypermobile, and that combined with all of the passive stretching while practicing and teaching yoga was one of the primary culprits for my discomfort. Initially I tried more passive, alternative healing modalities, such as Rolfing, acupuncture, and massage, to relieve my pain. However, it was ultimately dedicated physical therapy appointments and studying kinesiology, exercise science, and other forms of movement outside of yoga that helped me get off the pain hamster wheel.

My experience, education outside of traditional yoga, practice of Pilates on the apparatus, strength training, and somatic movement all helped me to understand the importance of cross training. I realized that only practicing asana and stretching was no longer serving me, but it could still be a part of my life and movement practice if I did other things as well. Over time, my pursuit of advanced education evolved into leading my own continuing education workshops to help other teachers better understand how to apply modern movement science concepts to their classes and personal movement practice to help themselves and their students. My personal experience combined with over a decade of working with private clients and providing continuing education courses for movement teachers has given me the insight to take what I've learned and condense it into this book.

This book is structured to show you how I teach my group classes and what the different parts of my classes look like. It also includes science-based information to explain why I structure the classes the way that I do, so you can understand why sequencing movements in this way may be helpful for students who have been injured and completed physical therapy, but are not ready to return to a traditional yoga class. What I've observed in my fifteen years of teaching is that many people are not sure where to start when returning to the yoga studio after experiencing pain or an injury. My hope is that this book acts as a guide for you to help your students return to regular exercise or movement, while maintaining your scope of practice as a yoga teacher.

In this book, you will learn somatic sequences, preparatory exercises, and principles of regression and progression to make your classes adaptable and appropriate for this post-rehab segment of the population. While there will never be a one-size-fits-all method for group classes, there are ways to structure your group classes that give people options, choices, and a pathway back to wellness, and this book has been written as a resource to help you guide your students on that path.

Trina Altman
Los Angeles, USA
August 2020

ACKNOWLEDGMENTS

Taking what I have learned as a yoga and movement teacher and using it to write a book has been one of the most challenging and rewarding experiences of my career. With that in mind, I need to extend my gratitude to the following people whose support and help made this book possible.

This book would not exist were it not for my friend and colleague Nikki Naab-Levy. Her linear thinking and journalism background helped me create a written framework to share my creativity and knowledge in a way that would be simple to follow and understand. Nikki, I can't tell you how much I appreciate your support through the process of bringing this book to life. Your problem-solving skills, deep knowledge of exercise science, attention to detail, and resourcefulness reduced the stress and challenges that I experienced as a writer.

This book would also not exist without the support of my husband, Farzad Rezai. Thank you for sacrificing our time together on the weekends so I could be at the computer writing. Beyond that, I am so appreciative of your endless encouragement that I pursue my interests and passions even when they were stressful, consuming, and at times impractical. It is because of you that I have felt the confidence to take on new, scary, and challenging endeavors like this for the past 17 years.

To my mother and father. Thank you for instilling a love of learning in me from an early age. Every time you brought me to an elementary school book club, gymnastics class, cheerleading practice, and summer camp activity, you provided me with an opportunity to figure out who I was and what brought me joy. You taught me the importance of never giving up even when things are hard and how to ask for help when a challenge seems impossible. These lessons allowed me to survive chemistry and trigonometry in my youth and have fueled my success as an adult. I am forever grateful to you for the life I have lived.

I also want to thank my mother-in-law Vida Shajie and father-in-law Feridoun Rezai, whom I am so fortunate to be able to call family. Vida, thank you so much for your encouragement that I pursue my interest in teaching yoga. Feridoun, I am so grateful for your love and support in my professional pursuits. You both mean the world to me.

This book would not have been possible without my teachers and mentors, who gave me the skills and confidence to develop my own voice as a teacher. Kim Valeri, thank you for giving me the gift of yoga. It was through my 200- and 300-hour teacher trainings with you that I discovered a new career path and found a way of living that I could finally call "home." Rise Karns Stockstad, thank you for giving me the gift of Pilates. Seeing you teach in a way that was smart, loving, and sustainable made me realize that it was possible to help myself and others through similar methods. Additionally, I want to express my appreciation to Marie-José Blom for showing me how teaching is both an art and a science. Being in your presence was an endless opportunity for me to learn and grow.

It would be remiss not to acknowledge several of my colleagues, many of whom I am also honored to call friends:

To Dana McCaw, thank you for setting an example of what it means to be a mentor and a colleague. Your kindness, patience, and work ethic have never failed to inspire me. I learned so much from you during our collaboration for Best Stretch Ever. Even as an experienced teacher, I gained an even deeper insight into how to sequence and create incredible classes, and I credit you for being the person who helped me overcome my fear of using PowerPoint.

To Madeline Black, Carrie Owerko, and Jules Mitchell, who embody what it means to be an incredible teacher and educator. Thank you for being examples of what is possible and for demonstrating how Pilates and yoga teachers can learn from outside disciplines and integrate what they learn to enhance the experience of students and teachers.

Thank you, Gil Hedley, for introducing me to the magic and wholeness of our bodies and creating a safe space to explore anatomy without fear or competition. And thanks go to Aline LaPierre, Anita Sawyer, and Janelle

ACKNOWLEDGMENTS

Railey for your kindness, support, and wisdom, which has given me strength in difficult times as a teacher.

To Andrew Serrano and Audrina Kingen, thank you for teaching me how to develop physical strength and showing me how it could foster greater physical and emotional resiliency. I extend my gratitude to Christopher Walling, Sarah Court, and Laurel Beversdorf for their friendship, wisdom, and support – thank you for being role models of how to blend academic brilliance with love and kindness. Additionally, thank you to June Chiang and Sean Hampton for helping me build a stronger foundation for movement, translating complicated verbiage into something I could understand and later teach, and for helping me manage my hypermobility.

I also thank the communities I have been blessed to be a part of, who paved the way for me to be able to write this book. To the STOTT PILATES®, Tune Up Fitness®, and Yogaspirit® communities, thank you for giving me lifelong friendships and endless opportunities to grow as a teacher and a person.

Finally, I thank my students. To the students in my Equinox classes, thank you for always being willing to join me on a new embodied adventure and consistently showing up with kindness and an eagerness to learn and explore. To my clients, thank you for teaching me through your questions and presence. It is through you that I've learned and experienced the healing power of human connection. Beyond that, you always remind me that movement is meant to be playful and fun. Barbara, you definitely have inspired an exercise name or two in this book!

Trina Altman
Los Angeles, USA
August 2020

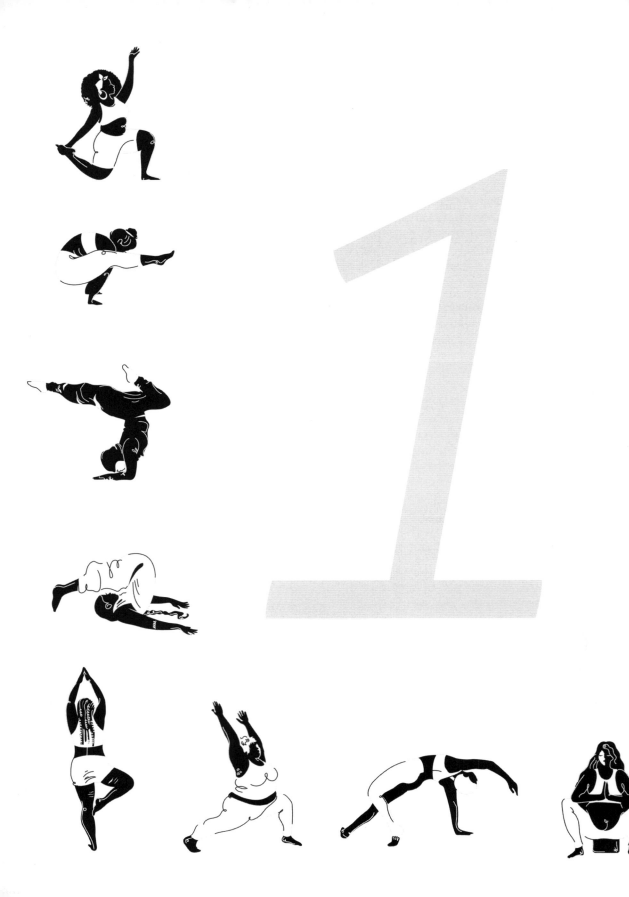

In the Western world, yoga has become a household name and a $16-billion industry (Yoga Alliance 2016) that is viewed by many as a natural or non-medical remedy for stress, pain, and trauma. It is also seen as a low-impact and joint-friendly form of exercise that can improve flexibility and be used as an alternative to going to the gym. Between 2012 and 2016, the number of Americans practicing yoga doubled. The 2016 Yoga in America Study conducted by *Yoga Journal* and Yoga Alliance estimated that 36 million Americans practiced yoga, and found that flexibility and stress were the primary reasons people gave for taking it up (Yoga Journal 2016).

However, despite the fact that people seek out yoga for its gentle and therapeutic reputation, many yoga teachers and students are injured as a result of practicing it. An epidemiology study published in the *Orthopedic Journal of Sports Medicine* observed that between 2001 and 2014, there were 29,590 yoga-related injuries reported to hospital emergency departments. The trunk was the most frequently injured area, and sprains and strains accounted for 45 percent of the injuries. The greatest number of injuries occurred among people who were aged 65 and older (Swain and McGwin 2016). This is noteworthy because the number of people over the age of 50 practicing yoga tripled between 2012 and 2016 (Yoga Journal 2016).

Given that yoga is recommended as a gentle and joint-friendly form of movement, it is important for us to consider why so many people are injured or develop pain when practicing it. We should also ask ourselves what we can do as teachers to reduce the risk of this happening in our classes.

Why do people get hurt doing yoga?

Assessing how and why an injury happens is complicated; multiple factors must be considered, including the individual circumstances of the injured person. However, most yoga injuries can be linked back to a single cause: how Western yoga classes are typically taught and the outdated belief system within yoga culture that perpetuates this method of teaching.

Here is an overview of some common causes of yoga injuries. Subsequent chapters in this book will cover some of what is mentioned below in greater depth.

Teacher consideration

Many students have an idealized version of a pose that they want to achieve. However, they may not fully understand the exercise progressions required to prepare their body for that pose and may try to force the position, even if they experience discomfort or signals from their body that it is not the best position for them in that moment. As you read this book, start to consider how you can create a sense of curiosity and appreciation for progressive movement and incremental progress instead of valuing practicing the most difficult-looking pose.

Modern postural yoga classes are not well designed for individuals in the modern world

Modern daily life rarely demands diverse and dynamic movement. The average person wakes up and sits at their kitchen table to eat breakfast. From there, they might sit in their car to drive to work, where they sit at a desk for hours. When they return home, they relax by sitting on their couch to watch TV. Even if they go to the gym, they will only have been active for a small portion of their day.

Modern movement science has found that the human body adapts to the loads and positions to which it is most frequently exposed. As a result, the average person is well adapted to sit, stand, and walk short distances. It is also now thought that injuries occur when a joint is loaded in a range that it is not well adapted for and does not have the strength to control. This is applicable to asana, because the average class in the Western world is taught as a series of poses that require loading a large amount of one's own bodyweight on to joints at their end ranges of motion. Given that the average person seldom, if ever, moves their joints to their end ranges of motion during daily life, it makes sense that doing so with little to no preparation when they begin a yoga practice might create the potential for injury. This could also explain why yoga injuries are so prevalent among older adults. The longer that an individual goes without loading their joints at the end ranges of motion, the weaker they will become in these ranges and the less prepared they will be to load their joints at the end ranges of motion during yoga practice. Beyond that, many people experience a steady decrease in strength as they age, so older adults could potentially have an increased risk of injury if they practice a movement for which they are not well prepared. A study published in the *Muscle, Ligaments and Tendons Journal* found that muscle strength declines between 16.6–40.9% for people between the ages of 40 and 80 (Keller and Engelhardt 2013). As a result, many of the individuals who come to our classes do not have the strength and movement skills required for the poses taught in a modern postural yoga class, which makes them vulnerable to injury. The solution to this is not to demonize traditional yoga poses, but to teach our students how to build strength through larger ranges of motion with a gradual increase in load over time. We can then better prepare them to practice yoga with a reduced risk of pain or injury.

Lack of cross training and external load

Pain or injury can also result from a lack of cross training and external loading when practicing yoga. Modern postural yoga is bodyweight training, which means the only option for loading is how much a person weighs. The majority of people who come to yoga are not strong enough to push their own bodyweight, and their joints are only prepared to tolerate the loads and directions of movement to which they have been regularly and progressively exposed. If someone loads their bodyweight on to a joint that is not well prepared to handle that load, it can result in injury.

This problem could be solved if modern postural yoga incorporated external loading, such as using dumbbells or resistance bands, allowing people to choose a level of resistance that their joints could safely tolerate. Over time, as their tissues became stronger and their joints adapted, people could choose heavier loads, until they were strong enough to train with their own bodyweight. In exercise science, this concept is known as progressive overload, which is defined as the gradual increase of stress placed upon a joint during exercise. Without the opportunity for progressive overload, most people's muscles and joints are underloaded for the demands of a typical yoga class.

Another issue with the lack of external loading in modern postural yoga is that there are no opportunities to load in the direction of pulling. If someone also cross trains, this would not be a problem. However, asana is often the only form of physical exercise that yoga teachers and students practice. Over time, this can lead to an imbalance, where students become stronger in the pushing directions of movement and weaker in the pulling directions of movement. So, tissues are not only generally underloaded to meet the physical demands of yoga, they are more underloaded in the direction of pulling, which can compound the risk of pain and injury.

Pain and injury can result from underloading or overloading a joint. One of the issues with only practicing yoga is that it can create a scenario for the joints to become underloaded and overloaded at the same time. This is because most yoga classes involve a high repetition of a limited number of movements. For example, many forms of modern postural yoga practice set sequences of poses without deviation, meaning that a single class could involve performing the same poses dozens of times. When these poses are practiced repetitively, it can result in a repetitive stress injury, where pain is experienced in the muscles, nerves, and tendons as a result of overuse through repetitive movement. The ideal solution to reduce incidences of pain and injury from under- and overloading would be for yoga practitioners to include cross training using external resistance, such as strength training or Pilates exercises on the apparatuses. However, many students are resistant to going to the gym or performing exercise on their own. Instead, we can incorporate external load and pulling movements into our yoga classes to mitigate the negative effects of over- and underloading.

A check/recheck is any technique that can be used to self-assess changes in your body when practicing a sequence. Check/rechecks can apply to any type of sequence, including yoga poses, sensory feedback methods, somatic exercises, and preparatory exercises. Changes that you can assess for include range of motion, breath capacity, strength, emotional state, and positional awareness.

Exploration of external load and pulling movements

1. Triangle Pose with resistance band from underneath bottom foot to top hand

Check: Come into Triangle Pose. Step your feet about three- to four-feet apart. Turn your right foot out and your left foot in. Reach your arms out to the side horizontally at shoulder height. Move into deeper flexion at the right hip as you reach your right hand down and place it on your shin or a yoga block. Reach your left arm straight up to the ceiling. Notice how it feels.

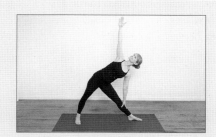
Triangle Pose check

Triangle Pose with a resistance band: Repeat the actions in regular Triangle Pose above, but use a resistance band by placing it underneath your right foot and holding it in your left hand. Or tie loops at either end of the band and put it around your right foot and left hand.

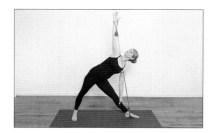
Triangle Pose with a resistance band

Recheck: Come into Triangle Pose. Notice how it may feel different after using the resistance bands. Did it feel easier to maintain muscular activation in the pose? Were there aspects of the pose that you couldn't sense before that you can sense now, and if so, what were they? Do you still feel like you need to place weight into your bottom hand to sustain the pose?

2. Blanket on back of head and upper thoracic spine in plank

Check: Come into Plank Pose and sense the position of your rib cage, spine, and head. Can you sense where your head is relative to your spine? Can you sense where your shoulder blades are relative to your spine and rib cage without looking in a mirror?

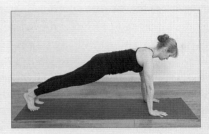

Plank Pose

Resume Plank Pose with a folded blanket resting on the back of your head and upper back. Notice if the feedback from the weight of the blanket helps you sense the position of your head and thorax.

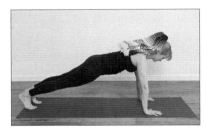

Plank Pose with a blanket

Recheck: Come into Plank Pose one more time without the blanket. Notice if it is easier to sense where your head, spine, rib cage, and shoulder blades are relative to one another. Often it is easy to sink in the rib cage or drop the head in Plank Pose. Notice if having the blanket as proprioceptive feedback and external resistance made it easier to find the muscular activation required to hold this pose.

3. Dandasana stretchy band rows

Check: Come into Plank Pose and slowly lower yourself onto your belly. As you bend your elbows, think about pulling yourself towards the floor and retracting your shoulder blades.

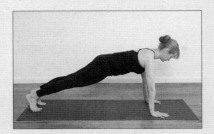

Dandasana stretchy band rows check

Dandasana with mid rows: Come into Dandasana with a resistance band looped around the bottom of your feet, one loop in each hand. Check that when your arms are straight you still have tension in the band. Slowly bend your elbows and pull the band towards you, while squeezing your shoulder blades together to activate the muscles in your upper and mid back.

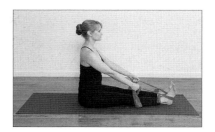

Dandasana stretchy band rows elbows straight

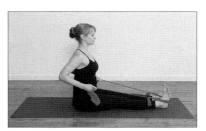

Dandasana stretchy band rows elbows bent

Recheck: Resume Plank Pose and slowly lower yourself onto your belly. Is it easier to come down in one piece rather than collapsing in one area of your torso, such as the pelvis, rib cage, or spine, after integrating your pulling muscles into the exercise?

Teacher consideration

Often after class, students ask questions about how to address overuse injuries or discomfort as a result of their yoga practice. In this scenario, it can be helpful to have a response prepared. If you are asked this question, how might you respond? For example, you could explain to them how cross training may be beneficial for their yoga practice. What other things might you say?

Competitive culture

The marketing and beliefs around yoga in the Western world are confusing and at times conflicting. On one hand, it is viewed as a gentle and therapeutic mind–body practice, which medical professionals recommend to their patients to reduce stress and alleviate pain. At the same time, it is represented on the covers of magazines and by social media influencers as a practice that allows the performance of impressive feats of flexibility and strength in the form of backbends, arm balances, and handstands, preferably on a beach with the perfect tan. These images are often accompanied by testaments to how yoga can help reduce anxiety, free us from self-judgment, achieve optimal health, and become our best selves. Becoming a more evolved person while mastering impossible-looking poses is a compelling sales pitch, especially in a society that rewards a perceived mastery of one's body and mind. No wonder yoga has become so popular.

Beyond that, many people who seek out yoga to reduce stress are high achievers with a competitive streak who operate with the mindset that more is better. As a result, they are likely to choose classes that emphasize the performative aspects of the practice. Even if a person doesn't have a desire to master advanced poses, they have likely heard the conventional wisdom that if something hurts, you should stretch it, and that increasing flexibility will help eliminate tension and pain. Since yoga is associated with increasing flexibility, it is an obvious choice for someone who is looking for a natural solution to addressing pain or discomfort.

When combined, these factors create a scenario where students have a preconceived notion of what their experience in a yoga class should entail before they ever step inside a studio. Since they've seen the poses in the media and heard about why yoga is good for you, they have predetermined expectations about what they should be learning in a class, a belief system around the right way to practice a pose, and often a specific goal in mind, which for the majority of people is to increase flexibility to minimize pain and tension, achieve difficult-looking poses, and reduce stress, preferably all at the same time.

There's nothing inherently wrong with the desire to master acrobatic poses or become more flexible. However, students are often compelled to attempt the most advanced version of a pose and stretch to their furthest limits, instead of adjusting their movements based on how it feels. This can also create a need to chase a sensation by going as deep as possible into a pose. While this can cause issues for people with any level of flexibility, it can be particularly problematic for hypermobile students who won't feel anything until they have moved into extreme ranges of motion, which can feel good in the moment but may contribute to joint instability and pain in the future. Furthermore, many students have been taught that pain is a normal part of the process and that if they practice long enough the pain will go away. This causes them to push through any warning signs that they may experience until the discomfort has escalated into an injury or a level of pain that can no longer be ignored.

This dynamic can be particularly challenging for yoga teachers. While they seek to build a sustainable practice using their understanding of how to prepare the joints for challenging poses in a way that minimizes the risk of pain and injury, their students might demand a certain type of pose or pacing based on their expectation of what yoga is supposed to look like. One of my hopes in writing this book is to give you a framework for teaching that is educational and empowering, and provides your students with an element of what they expect while minimizing their risk of pain and injury.

Hands-on assists

Many yoga teacher trainings include hands-on assists for yoga poses. While touch can be therapeutic in the right setting, it can be problematic in the yoga space. One issue is how hands-on assists are performed. Many hands-on assists in yoga involve pushing the body into extreme ranges of motion with force. For some students, any amount of force can feel like too much, for others, heavy amounts of force might feel good in the moment but could result in pain and even injury later.

Also, in a group class setting, teachers usually do not know the physical or mental health histories of their students. Without this history and the time to work with each student privately, teachers cannot know if a student has physical issues where adjustments are contraindicated. Furthermore, many individuals do not feel comfortable disclosing their mental health history to take a yoga class, and they shouldn't be required to. For some individuals, any unexpected or unsolicited touch can be traumatizing, particularly if an individual has a history of trauma. For individuals with trauma, they may consent to touch, even if they don't actually want it, and they may experience an adverse reaction to being touched. A research article published in *Depression and Anxiety* in 2019 looked at two studies that analyzed the experience and neural processing of interpersonal and impersonal touch with people who had been diagnosed with post-traumatic stress disorder (PTSD) as compared to people without a history of trauma. The studies concluded that while people without a history of trauma appreciated touch, individuals with a history of PTSD disliked it. This was also reflected in neural activation. The study found that for individuals with PTSD, hippocampal suppression occurred as an attempt to control traumatic memories that were evoked by touch and that this mechanism may maintain the aversion of interpersonal touch in patients with interpersonal trauma-related PTSD (Strauss et al. 2019). Even if they do not have a history of trauma, many students who attend a yoga class expect it to be similar to a group fitness class, where the teacher stands at the front of the room and instructs the class. In this situation, they will not attend class expecting to be adjusted, and may find being touched uncomfortable and an invasion of their personal space.

Beyond that, for many yoga teachers, hands-on assists go beyond their scope of practice. This is particularly relevant in the United States, where many states have laws that require a license to touch a client and specific education to legally be able to perform any type of adjustment involving stretching or moving another person's body. Some professions with a license to touch include physical therapy, medicine, chiropractic, and massage therapy. In a broad sense, if you perform hands-on adjustments without the appropriate license and education, the laws of your state might interpret that action as practicing medicine without a license. With all of this in mind, a simple way to stay within your scope of practice and reduce the risk of injury in a group yoga class is to avoid hands-on assists when you are teaching.

A way to provide proprioceptive feedback to the body in a class setting without a hands-on assist is to use a prop.

Examples of how to use props in place of hands-on assists

1. Using a yoga block to provide tactile feedback in Plank Pose

If you are teaching Plank Pose, you can invite your students to place a yoga block horizontally across their shoulder blades and have them protract and retract their shoulder blades in this position. The weight of the yoga block will allow them to sense when they move into protraction that their spine comes into greater contact with the block, and when they move into retraction, their spine moves away from the block. In this scenario, the block replaces a hands-on assist that you might apply to the upper back between the shoulder blades to help your students notice what it is like to activate the muscles of their upper back to help support their joints in Plank Pose.

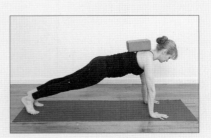

Scapular protraction in Plank Pose

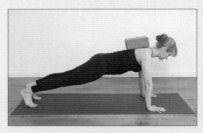

Scapular retraction in Plank Pose

2. Using a yoga strap under the mid back when in supine to provide feedback to the positioning of the ribs

A common tendency during supine core exercises, such as dead bug, is to bring the mid back into spinal extension by lifting the base of the rib cage off the floor, which makes it difficult to sense the activation of the abdominal muscles. Since many students will be unaware that they are extending through the mid or lower back, it is beneficial to offer tactile feedback. In a private session, you could place your fingertips underneath the part of your student's spine that is moving into extension. However, you could achieve a similar result in a class setting by first inviting students to find a partner. From there, one person would lie supine with a yoga strap on the floor positioned horizontally just below the inferior angle of the shoulder blades. You could then ask them to press that area of their back into the strap, so their partner is unable to pull the strap away. To minimize strain or hyperextension in the cervical spine, you may also need to place a blanket underneath the head and upper back.

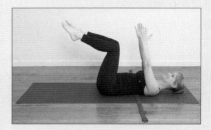

Yoga strap under mid back in supine

3. Using a block behind the pelvis to provide tactile feedback to pelvic positioning during side-lying movements

A common compensation in side-lying bent-knee hip circles is for the pelvis to roll backwards, which bypasses using hip muscles to create controlled circumduction at the hip joint. A hands-on strategy to address this might be to stand behind your student with your shin bone against their sacrum, so they can feel if their hip rolls back. A way to mimic this assist would be to invite them to place a yoga block behind their buttocks and instruct them to practice the movement without knocking the block over.

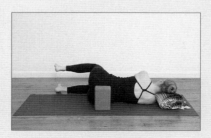

Block behind pelvis in side lying

Teacher consideration

Consider your own thoughts and experiences with hands-on assists. Do you like or dislike them? Have you found them to be harmful or helpful? Do you believe that they are appropriate in a private session, but not in a group class? Do you find them beneficial in a teacher training, but not in a class for the general public? Use this reflection to begin to develop your own policy around how you will approach hands-on assists when teaching, and your own preferences when taking classes in your personal practice.

Biomechanically incorrect cueing

Most yoga teacher trainings teach stylistic technique from a specific lineage, which means that the cues are usually not based on exercise science. As a result, many of the cues used in modern postural yoga contradict biomechanical principles about how joints are meant to move.

For example, a common yoga cue used for poses such as Warrior I and Downward Facing Dog is "pull your shoulders down." This will cause many people to aggressively depress their shoulder blades, instead of allowing for the natural scapulohumeral rhythm of upward rotation. While depressing the shoulder blades in overhead movements won't necessarily cause an injury, if practiced repeatedly it can create ongoing discomfort or irritation in the joint.

This is a single example of how an innocent cue can result in pain or an injury. However, there are numerous instances where this can happen at each of the joints. While yoga teachers don't need to have an advanced degree in exercise science to teach safe classes, it is beneficial to learn more about how joints are meant to move, so we can understand if the cues that we are using make biomechanical sense.

Exploration of upward rotation versus scapular depression with full shoulder flexion

Find a comfortable seated position and slowly reach your arms out in front of you and up to the ceiling. Pause when your upper arm bones are next to your ears. Can you sense the upward rotation of your shoulder blades in this position?

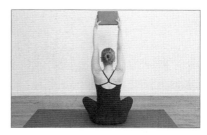

Full shoulder flexion with upward rotation

Repeat the same action. However, once your upper arm bones are next to your ears, depress your shoulder blades down towards the floor.

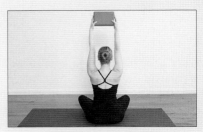

Full shoulder flexion with scapular depression

Can you sense how these two ways of moving into glenohumeral flexion involve different types of muscular engagement and placement of the scapulae?

Teacher consideration

Consider why you choose the cues that you use when teaching yoga. Do you use certain cues because you are repeating what you heard your teacher say in your yoga teaching training, or do you choose cues with the goal of helping a student learn a movement skill or better understand a movement that they are practicing? If you do have a favorite way to cue certain poses, do these cues seem to elicit more clarity or confusion for your students when you watch them move?

What is Yoga Deconstructed?

Yoga Deconstructed is an approach to teaching yoga that incorporates modern movement science in helping to prepare students for asana and activities of daily life. This teaching approach addresses some of the more common reasons why someone might experience pain or injury when practicing yoga. Yoga Deconstructed incorporates regressions, progressions, somatic movements, sensory feedback methods, and preparatory exercises to prepare the joints for asana and introduces external loads and pulling movements to reduce the risk of repetitive stress injuries. It also structures the class in a way that honors the experience of yoga, while teaching functional movement skills that make the practice more accessible and sustainable for students.

There is no rule that a yoga class must include functional movement skills. However, it is important to consider the benefits of unspecialized or functional movement and how these benefits relate to the motivation behind why many of our students come to yoga. While some students may want to learn how to do challenging arm balances or the splits, many people decide to try yoga because a medical professional recommended it to reduce stress or pain. Additionally, for many people, yoga is their only form of exercise, so a yoga class might be the one opportunity that they have to improve their movement fluency and resiliency. If a student is attending a yoga class with the primary goal of mastering challenging yoga poses, this approach can help them prepare for advanced poses, while reducing their risk of injury. Ultimately, incorporating these ideas into your teaching can better meet the needs of all your students regardless of their goals.

Yoga Deconstructed is different from most modern postural yoga classes both in the sequence and selection of the poses. Unlike a traditional vinyasa flow class, this approach incorporates external load through the use of props and a series of pose progressions and regressions to prepare the body for a sequence of peak poses. The result is a class designed around exercise science principles that promotes strength and resilience and builds the foundation for a lifelong yoga practice.

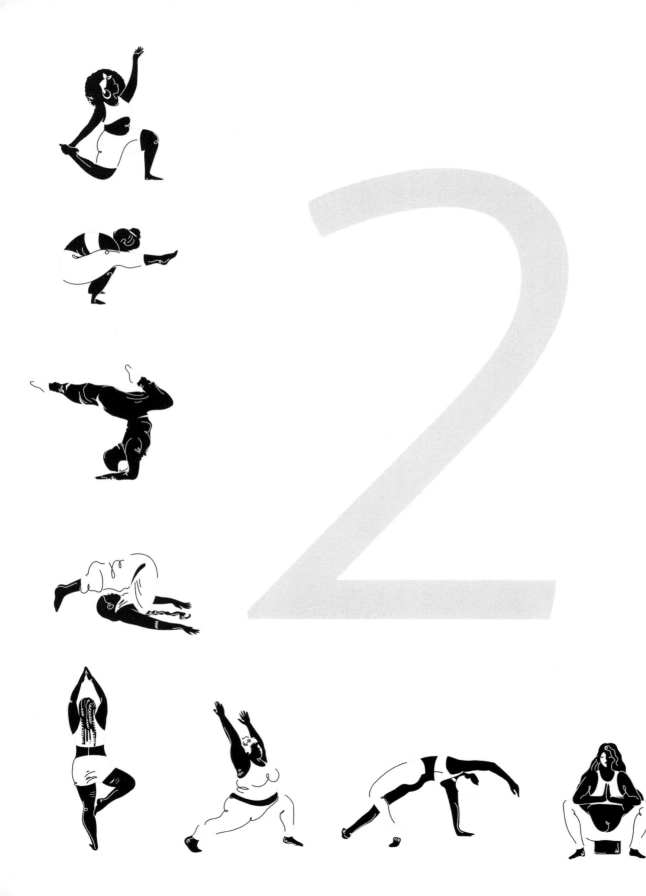

As movement teachers, we have a lot of options for which exercises and poses we choose to teach in our classes. As a result, deciding what to teach and in what sequence can become overwhelming, and so I find it is helpful to use the following principles to inform these decisions:

1. Total embodiment

2. Understanding the underlayer

3. Regress to progress

4. Creating an environment of safety

Principle 1: Total embodiment

Many modern postural yoga classes primarily rely on verbal cues to teach poses; the teacher walks around the room and verbally instructs students through sequences. If there are any demonstrations, they often occur near the end of the class for a handful of advanced poses. While verbal cueing is an essential tool for leading a class, this style of teaching relies primarily on only one mode of learning, which can make the class less accessible for students who don't absorb information well by listening.

Modes of learning are sets of guidelines that categorize how a person acquires, processes, and retains information. No one learns solely through a single mode, but many of us will learn better through some modes over others – it will depend on the individual. According to Rachel Zwass-Rupel, who holds a PhD in education from the UCLA Division of Human Development and Psychology, a teacher should employ as many modes of learning as possible to tap into people's strengths and increase their chances of making a tangible connection to what is being taught (Zwass-Rupel 2019). There are four primary modes or styles of learning: auditory, visual, reading/writing, and kinesthetic. Since reading and writing don't lend themselves well to teaching yoga, I will focus on the auditory, visual, and kinesthetic modes of learning here.

Auditory learning

Auditory learning is when a person takes in information by listening or speaking. In a yoga class, teaching with verbal cues would be the primary example of auditory learning. There are two types of cueing that you can use when teaching: internal cueing and external cueing. Internal cueing involves cueing the position of one body part relative to another or drawing awareness to a sensation, including quality of breath or the engagement of a specific muscle group. Some examples of internal cueing include:

- Reach your knees over your toes. (This is an internal cue, because you are cueing the position of one body part relative to another.)

- Engage your glutes to lift your hips. (This is an internal cue, because you are cueing a specific muscle group to initiate the movement.)

- Feel your thigh bone spiral outward as your shin bone spirals inward. (This is an internal cue, because you are cueing the position of one bone relative to another bone.)

Internal cueing can be beneficial for fostering proprioception, or body awareness, which in turn can improve motor control and coordination. If a student is new to movement, is returning after an injury, or has a history of pain, they may have limited proprioception and so internal cueing can be particularly helpful in these scenarios. Research suggests that internal cueing may assist in increasing muscle activation in specific areas of the body. An article published in the *Strength and Conditioning Journal* analyzed the results of several studies on the effects of internal cueing on muscle activation. It reported that in one study, participants were able to alter electromyography (EMG) activity in the rectus abdominis and obliques when verbally instructed to focus on activating one of the two muscle groups while practicing a curl up. Another study found that participants were able to achieve greater EMG activity in the gluteus maximus with decreased hamstring engagement when they were instructed to contract their glutes and keep the hamstrings relaxed during prone hip extension exercises (Schoenfeld and Contreras 2016). While the idea of increased muscle engagement has historically been used as a way for bodybuilders to increase muscle size, this strategy can also help students who struggle with proprioceptive awareness, because it allows them to focus on what they are engaging and feel more stable during movement. This can be especially beneficial for hypermobile students, who will often struggle to feel muscle engagement in the areas where they are hypermobile.

External cueing occurs when you cue something outside of the body or give a student a focal point outside of themselves. When teaching movement, external cueing often takes place in the form of instructing the directionality of a movement or giving the student a task to complete. Examples of external cueing include:

- Point your toes towards the front of the room. (This is an external cue, because it is task based and involves orienting the student in a specific direction towards something outside of themselves.)

- Stand in Warrior II and rip the mat apart with your feet. (This is an external cue, because the student has been given a task to complete. Note how this will create a sense of muscular engagement in the hip abductors without having to cue a specific muscle group.)

- Pass the yoga block from hand to hand. (This cue, which could be used when someone is in Locust Pose, is an external cue, because the student has been given the task of passing the yoga block.)

External cueing is beneficial for learning skills and improving motor performance. In the case of yoga, it can be used to refine the execution of a pose or improve balance. An article published in the *International Review of Sport and Exercise Psychology* analyzed research conducted over 15 years on attentional focus (another term for external cueing), and motor performance. The article reported that providing an external focus improved accuracy and consistency of movement, balance, efficiency, muscular activity, and force production (Wulf 2013).

External cueing can also be helpful for students with pain and hyperawareness around how movement affects the area that hurts. Giving them an external task allows them to direct their attention towards what they are doing, instead of fixating on the area in pain. In many cases, this can reduce the fear or guarding response that sometimes occurs when someone expects a movement to be painful. For instance, if a student expects to experience shoulder pain when they reach their arm overhead, it is more likely that their shoulder will hurt when they consciously make that movement. However, if instructed to reach for a yoga block and this happens to require overhead movement, it is less likely that they'll notice discomfort, or they may be able to move through a greater range of motion before the discomfort occurs.

Applying internal and external cueing to yoga

When considering how to best cue a yoga class, it is important to note that one type of cueing isn't better than the other. Rather, you want to consider why you are choosing to cue a pose in a certain way.

Internal cueing can help your students sense and feel where they are in space. It can also help them become aware of what they are feeling and how they are moving. This can be useful if you want to draw their attention to a specific area of the body to refine a movement pattern or notice how a style of breathing or a position feels. However, internal cueing can also be confusing and disorienting, especially if a student is unfamiliar with a pose or anatomical jargon. For instance, if someone has difficulty balancing and doesn't have very much awareness of the position of their knee and hip joints, then cueing them to spiral their thigh bone relative to their shin bone while also trying to remain upright in a challenging position can result in frustration. Additionally, internal cueing may not be ideal for students who have pain or heightened sensitivity around a specific area of their body, because it may cause them to micromanage or become fearful of a movement if they sense any discomfort.

Conversely, external cueing can be helpful for creating more organic and functional muscular engagement. For instance, instructing a student to "rip the mat apart" when in a wide-legged stance can cause the muscles around the hips to engage and stabilize the pelvis. In many ways, this is more practical than instructing a student to "squeeze their glutes," because it results in all the muscles of the legs engaging without the student having to think about it. Similarly, instructing a student to aim for a yoga block or to avoid knocking over a yoga block can give them a more concrete sense of where they are in space, because they have immediate feedback from the environment around them. This is one reason why props are so beneficial when teaching yoga. However, external cues can become more powerful when combined with internal cues because of the enhanced proprioceptive awareness.

For example, maybe you want to help your students refine their execution of Bird Dog. In this scenario, you could use a combination of internal and external cues. You might initially set them up for the movement with:

- Come onto your hands and knees with your hips over your knees and your shoulders over your hands (internal cue).

- Stack two or three blocks just outside of your left thigh (external cue).

- Push your hands into the ground (external cue) and spread your shoulder blades away from your spine (internal cue).

- Reach your left hand to the wall in front of you and your right leg to the wall behind you (external cue).

- Try not to knock the blocks over with your left hip or leg (external cue).

- Pause in this position and see if you can hold your head, ribs, and pelvis in one long line (internal cue).

- Lower your hand and foot to the ground with control (external cue).

Notice how in this scenario a combination of both internal and external cues was used to give students positional awareness of individual joints and their surroundings. Additionally, students were given a series of tasks to complete.

Each student will respond differently to your cues based on their history and interpretation of your words. Providing both internal and external cueing when teaching gives students the best opportunity to understand and follow your instructions. Remember, there is no right or wrong way to cue – the important thing is to stay adaptable and to adjust how you cue based on how your students respond.

Teacher consideration

Below is an example of how one might cue Warrior II. Can you identify which of these cues are internal cues and which are external cues?

1. Pick up your right foot and step it four feet away from your left foot with your toes parallel to each other.

2. Turn your right foot out to face the front of the room.

3. Reach your arms out to your sides, so they are horizontal to the ground.

4. Bend your right knee, so it lines up with roughly your second right toe.

5. Scrape your right heel backwards towards the back of the mat.

6. At the same time, scrape the inner edge of your left heel towards your right heel to activate your internal rotators and adductors.

Chapter 2

Visual learning

Visual learning is when someone learns through seeing something. In a classroom, this might include the use of visual aids, such as charts or diagrams. However, in a yoga class the primary mode of visual learning would be watching a teacher demonstrate a pose. Demonstrations are helpful because many students will struggle to understand yoga poses through only verbal cues. This is especially important if a pose or exercise is new to your students. Since it is likely that even an experienced yoga student will be new to some of the topics addressed in this book, such as preparatory exercises, somatic movements, creative use of props, and progressions or regressions, you will want to include visual demonstrations if you decide to incorporate these movements into your classes. However, it can be beneficial to demonstrate all modern postural yoga poses to meet the needs of visual learners and students who are new to class.

While it often makes sense to demonstrate at the front of the room, if you are teaching a sequence that is new to your students, you may want to have them gather in a circle around you to watch you demonstrate and allow everyone to see what is happening. This strategy also works well if the exercises that you are teaching take place on the floor and involve small movements, which can be difficult to see from the back of the room. This will apply to many preparatory exercises and

sensory feedback methods. You will also want to consider incorporating visual demonstrations if you are teaching an exercise with props, because many students will be confused by verbal cues that involve orienting them in a direction relative to a specific joint or body part. One more visual aid to consider using is a model skeleton, if the studio where you teach has one. A skeleton can help your students visualize the joints and the corresponding movements that you are cueing.

Kinesthetic learning

Kinesthetic learning occurs when a person learns by feeling or trying something. In yoga, one example of kinesthetic learning is when a student, through repetition, develops a feeling for the internal experience of practicing a pose. However, kinesthetic learning can also be enhanced by touch from an instructor or receiving tactile feedback from a prop, a wall, or the floor.

Since many yoga teachers do not have a license to touch (as is legally required in several states), it may be beyond your scope of practice to perform hands-on cueing or assists. And as previously mentioned, it is unlikely that you have a comprehensive mental health and physical history of the students in your class to ensure touch is appropriate for them. As a result, I recommend relying on props and the external environment for incorporating kinesthetic learning into your classes.

How to use props and the external environment for kinesthetic learning

One of the simplest things you can do to promote kinesthetic learning is to teach exercises where several parts of the body are in contact with the floor. This will typically apply to somatic and preparatory exercises, which take place in a side-lying, supine, or prone position.

If your students are in a supine position for a pose, you can draw their attention to how their shoulder blades, spine, ribs, and pelvis connect with the ground. Similarly, if your students are in a side-lying position, you can invite them to notice how one side of their body rests into the floor. If they are prone, you can ask them to notice how the front of their chest, abdomen, pelvis, and legs connect to the floor. Breath can also be a useful tool to promote kinesthetic awareness, because students can sense how it will cause areas of the body to become heavier or lighter on the ground as they inhale and exhale.

Another way to use your external environment for kinesthetic learning is to teach exercises that include feedback from the walls. This might include placing one or both hands or feet, or one side of the body, against the wall during exercises and poses such as Bird Dog, dead bug, side-lying leg lifts, or Warrior III.

You can also invite your students to touch areas of their body with their hands for kinesthetic feedback. Examples of this include placing the hands on the ribs, pelvis, or abdomen during exercises in supine and side lying. This strategy can be used to help your students understand how their breath affects their movement. It can also help your students learn how to differentiate movements: for example, if you were teaching how to differentiate movement between the pelvis and thigh bones, you could invite your students to place their hands on the front of the pelvis on the anterior superior iliac spines and notice how the pelvis posteriorly and anteriorly tilts while the thigh bones remain still. Keeping this hand placement and alternately lifting and lowering each leg to tabletop allows students to feel how the thigh bones can move independently of the pelvis.

Hands-on touch can also be used in conjunction with feedback from the floor or wall, which would allow your students to kinesthetically sense multiple sides of their body at once. For example, if you were teaching constructive rest, you could have your students place one hand on the sternum and the other hand on the abdomen. You could then invite them to sense how the back of the body connects to the floor, while also noticing how their chest and abdomen move towards their hands while inhaling.

Exploration of using your hands to enhance kinesthetic awareness

Lie on your back with your knees bent. Make a half-prayer position with your right hand and place your thumb at your sternum.

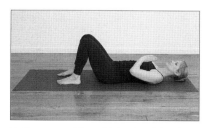

Half-prayer position with hand and thumb on sternum

Hold your sternum and rib cage still as you slowly sway your knees to the right. Bring your knees back to center.

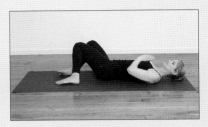

Knee sway to the right

Continue to hold your upper body still as you sway your knees to the left. Notice how this creates spinal rotation.

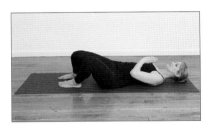

Knee sway to the left

Repeat the same movement, but as your knees sway to the right, allow your sternum and rib cage to roll to the right. Notice how this creates rolling instead of twisting.

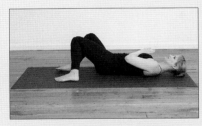

Knees, sternum, and ribcage rolling in the same direction

Can you sense how in the first version your shoulder blades and rib cage stayed in contact with the floor, whereas in the second example your left shoulder blade and the left side of your rib cage lost contact with the ground?

This exercise illustrates how you can guide your students to use their own hands to sense which parts of their body are moving and which parts are stable, and in this example, teaches them how to understand the difference between twisting and rolling. This strategy can replace a hands-on assist from the teacher.

Therapy balls are another beneficial tool for promoting kinesthetic learning, because they provide specific tactile feedback to areas of the body and nearby joints that students may have difficulty sensing or conceptualizing. While therapy balls can be used to provide feedback to many body parts, they can be particularly helpful for students to understand and sense areas of their body and joints that they can't see and have problems feeling. This is most applicable to the posterior side of the body, which includes the shoulder blades, thoracic spine, lumbar spine, and back of the pelvis.

I also recommend using props such as blankets, stretchy bands, and yoga blocks to incorporate kinesthetic learning into your classes, because the options they provide are endless. For example, below are three different ways that you could use yoga blocks to promote kinesthetic learning when teaching the preparatory exercise Bird Dog.

- Practice Bird Dog with a yoga block balanced on the sacrum, which will help your students sense where their pelvis is in space and may allow them to self-correct any lateral shifting or rotation in the pelvis.

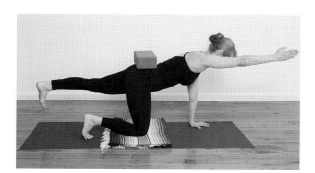

Bird Dog with block on sacrum

- Hold a yoga block when reaching the arm overhead, which will help your students sense the muscles around the shoulder girdle.

- Stack three yoga blocks next to the left thigh and instruct your students to extend the right leg without knocking the blocks over. This will give them feedback on the lateral aspect of their left thigh, which will help them sense any lateral shifting that may occur during the movement.

Some additional examples of how to use props for kinesthetic learning include:

- Practice Cat Cow with a resistance band near the thoracolumbar junction and one end of the band affixed at each hand to provide proprioceptive feedback to the back of the rib cage.

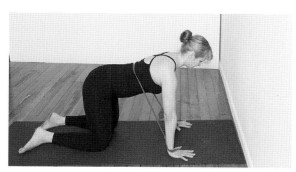

Cat Cow with band neutral spine

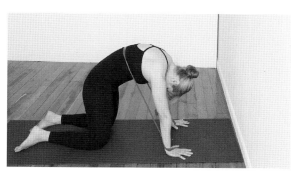

Cat Cow with band spinal flexion

Chapter 2

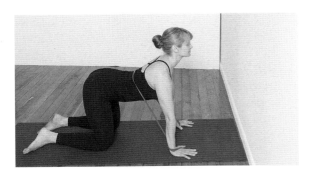

Cat Cow with band spinal extension

- Stand in Tadasana and walk around the room with a blanket and yoga block balanced on top of your head to sense head carriage.
- Place a rolled-up blanket between the thighs while practicing Chair Pose to kinesthetically sense the midline of the body.

Teacher consideration

Think of an exercise or pose that you often teach in classes. What are three different ways that you could incorporate kinesthetic learning?

In summary, the most effective way to help your students learn is to employ elements of each of these learning modes while teaching your classes. In terms of practical application, this would mean including a combination of internal and external verbal cues, physical demonstration, and using props for kinesthetic feedback in each class. This approach encourages a deeper understanding of the material and will allow each student to process new information through their preferred methods of learning.

Teacher consideration

Now that you are familiar with the different learning modes, consider how you learn best. Are you primarily a visual, kinesthetic, or auditory learner, or a combination of all three? Which modes of learning do you use most when teaching and why? What are some ways that you could incorporate other modes of learning into your classes?

Principle 2: Understanding the underlayer

Anatomical language and human movement can be confusing for teachers and students alike. Each individual steps onto their mat with a unique movement background, understanding, and language. As a result, no two people will interpret or experience cues and poses the same way. Additionally, the average yoga student does not have extensive movement education or body awareness, because these topics are not taught in school nor needed for most careers. This is why taking time at the beginning of class to explain the primary joints and joint-specific movements that you will be focusing on (the 'underlayer') can help your students understand the purpose of the exercises and cues that you use later in class.

As already discussed, individuals learn best when multiple learning modalities are incorporated when teaching. I advocate using this approach to help your students understand and sense where their joints are in space and how movement occurs at these joints. Since we have hundreds of joints and it would be impossible to cover all of them in a single class, I will often pick a theme or focus for each class. Below is my process for creating a class and choosing a class emphasis:

- Select a peak pose that I want to create the class around.

- List the directions of movement and joint mobility required for the peak pose.

- Use this list to pick an area of the body to focus on in class.

- Choose a series of exercises based on the directions of movement that progress to the peak pose and relate to the area of focus.

- Plan how I want to introduce the area of focus to my students at the beginning of class using somatic exercises or sensory feedback techniques, which will be discussed in later chapters.

Once I have identified the area of focus, I will consider how to incorporate different learning modalities, including auditory, kinesthetic, and visual cues to teach my students about that area.

Here is a simple way of helping your students have a more embodied and clear understanding of specific joints:

- Tell students what the area of focus is, and that it will be explained to them now so they have a better understanding of the cues and exercises that will come up later in class.

- Point to that area on yourself and use anatomical language and cues to describe it.

- Tell them the directions of movement for this joint and give an example of how these movements are helpful for activities of daily life.

- Invite students to feel that area on themselves using their hands or feedback from the floor or a prop.

An embodied approach to teaching ankle inversion and eversion

Side Plank is a common pose that many students struggle with, because they are not well prepared for the ankle movements required to practice the pose. Additionally, they may not understand how to move their ankles to comfortably assume the pose. Below is an example of how I might introduce the movements required for Plank Pose to help my students understand the underlayer, and to feel successful when they attempt Side Plank later in class.

1. Standing exploration of ankle inversion and eversion

Stand with your feet a comfortable distance apart.

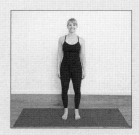

Standing exploration of ankle inversion starting position

Slowly peel the inner edges of your feet off the floor, so you are standing on the outer edges of your feet. This is called inversion of the ankle.

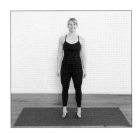

Ankle inversion

If this feels okay, you can increase the load by walking while maintaining ankle inversion.

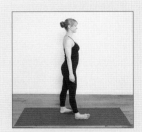

Ankle inversion with walking

Return to the starting position.

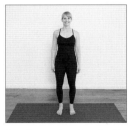

Standing exploration of ankle eversion starting position

Slowly peel the outer edges of your feet off the floor, so you are standing on the inner edges of your feet. This is called eversion of the ankle.

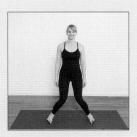

Ankle eversion

If this feels okay, you can increase the load by walking while maintaining ankle eversion. Note that for this movement exploration you will want to internally rotate your femurs and bend your knees.

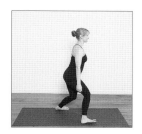

Ankle eversion with walking

This is an example of how you can progressively load your ankles in an inverted position and everted position, so they are better prepared for the ankle inversion and eversion that will happen when you teach Side Plank later in class. You can also think of this as an exercise regression for the ankles in Side Plank, which requires moving through ankle inversion, but has the additional challenge of balance and control through the upper body and spine.

2. Ankle inversion and eversion with a therapy ball

Place a therapy ball underneath the ball of your right foot while standing and keep your heel bone in contact with the ground. Roll the ball side to side. It should move across the metatarsophalangeal joints from the base of your big toe to the base of your pinky toe and back again.

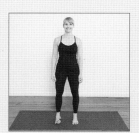

Ankle inversion with ball

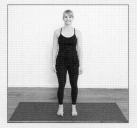

Ankle eversion with ball

This rolling action creates ankle inversion and eversion with proprioceptive feedback from the therapy ball. It also helps mobilize the ankle joint in dorsiflexion, so the ankles are better prepared not only for Side Plank, but other poses that you might teach later in class that require ankle dorsiflexion, such as Downward Facing Dog.

3. Check mark bridge with an emphasis on ankle eversion

Stack two blocks at the front edge of your mat on the lowest level. Lie on your back with your right knee bent and your left knee extended. Place the outer edge of your left foot on the top of the highest block. Notice how this causes your pelvis to rotate to the left and your right buttock to become light on the floor.

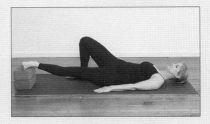

Check mark bridge starting position

Press both arms and your right foot into the floor to lift your pelvis in the air while strongly everting your left ankle.

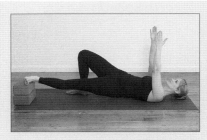

Check mark bridge with pelvis in the air

To increase the challenge, lift your arms off the floor.

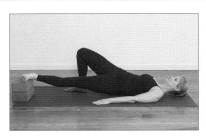

Check mark bridge with arms lifted off of the floor

You can add further challenge by lifting your left foot off the floor into a tabletop position.

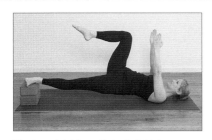

Check mark bridge with leg in tabletop

4. Progressively introduce ankle inversion and eversion in Side Plank

Come into Plank Pose with your feet shoulder-distance apart. Drop your head towards the floor, so you can see your feet.

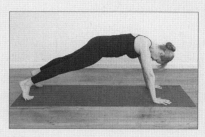

Plank Pose looking at feet

Dorsiflex your ankles and roll onto the inner edge of your left foot and the outer edge of your right foot until your left ankle is strongly everted and your right ankle is strongly inverted. Reverse directions and roll onto the inner edge of your right foot and the outer edge of your left foot to experience ankle inversion and eversion on the second side.

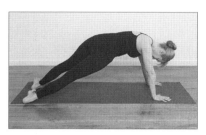

Plank Pose with ankle inversion and eversion

Next, place the inner edge of your left foot on top of the inner edge of your right foot. Lift your left arm up to the ceiling to come into a traditional Side Plank.

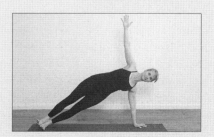

Traditional Side Plank

Can you sense how walking in inversion and eversion and the check mark bridge informed how you engage the muscles surrounding your ankles in Side Plank?

Chapter 2

Principle 3: Regress to progress

In modern postural yoga classes, students who experience pain or are unable to do a pose are often instructed to avoid the pose entirely or practice a modification with the aid of props to passively support their joints. While modifications can be beneficial, this approach fails to address the underlying reasons why a pose might be inaccessible and won't necessarily prepare someone to successfully practice it in the future. This can be remedied through the training principle of progression, which provides the critical thinking skills to create sequences that prepare the joints for more advanced poses with a reduced risk of pain and injury. This way of teaching can also increase your students' functionality and movement potential in and out of the classroom.

The training principle of progression is based on the idea that as the body adapts to a movement, you will need to gradually increase the overload or level of challenge to improve or develop a skill. However, these progressions must be incremental to prevent overloading the body's ability to recover. This is done by selecting a version of the exercise that is appropriate for the student's current level of strength and control. These versions of an exercise are often referred to as progressions and regressions. An exercise progression requires greater coordination and the control of more body parts simultaneously. An exercise regression lessens the stimulus, so a student can focus on a specific body part or single aspect of a movement. When choosing a progression or regression, you want to select an exercise that challenges a student's movement skills, but is not so difficult that they lose control.

To put this into the context of yoga, we must first consider how we define a yoga pose. While there is a lot that can be discussed on this subject, this section is going to define yoga poses as shapes that we can create with our body that have specific types of alignment. A progression in the context of yoga can be defined as when it is more challenging to maintain the alignment of a yoga pose or shape. A regression can be defined as when it is less challenging to maintain the alignment of a yoga pose or shape. Some yoga poses lend themselves to a variety of progressions and regressions, while others may have only one or two. However, understanding the factors involved in progression and regression will allow you to deconstruct any yoga pose.

Factors to consider when progressing or regressing a yoga pose

Load

The first factor to consider when progressing or regressing a pose is load, defined as the force exerted on the body. An increase in load will make the pose more challenging, and a decrease in load will make a pose less challenging. To summarize, load can be increased to progress a pose or decreased to regress a pose.

Another consideration is the type of load involved: internal or external. They are also sometimes referred to as intrinsic and extrinsic load, respectively. For the purposes of progressing or regressing a yoga pose, internal load can be thought of as a person's bodyweight, whereas external load can be any load or resistance that is independent of the person, such as a resistance band, free weight, or cork yoga block.

Both internal and external loads can be used to progress or regress a yoga pose. Internal load can be adjusted by placing more or less of one's bodyweight over a set of joints. For example, keeping the knees on the floor in Plank Pose would regress the pose, because less bodyweight would be centered over the wrists. Adding or taking away a prop is a way to progress or regress a yoga pose through external load. For instance, a simple progression of Warrior II would be to practice the pose while holding two cork blocks. A regression would be to practice the same pose without any blocks. This is because the cork blocks increase the amount of work required for a person to hold up their arms.

Exploring load in Setu Bandhasana

Check: Come into Setu Bandhasana. Are you able to sense the contraction of your glutes and hamstrings in this pose or are you more aware of the engagement of your spinal extensors?

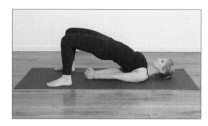

Setu Bandhasana check

Banded Setu Bandhasana: Lie down on your back with your knees bent and your feet flat on the floor. Place a resistance band across the front of your hip creases. Keep it connected to the floor and taut across your hips by placing your hands in a loop on each end of the band.

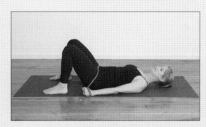

Banded Setu Bandasana starting position

Press your pelvis up towards the ceiling to create hip extension.

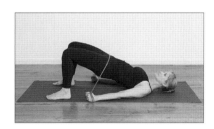

Banded Setu Bandasana with pelvis lifted

Lower with control. Notice how the external load of the resistance band causes your glutes and hamstrings to engage more than they did in the original pose.

Recheck: Come into Setu Bandhasana without the resistance band. Notice if it is easier to sense the activation of your glutes and hamstrings after adding external load with a resistance band.

27

Chapter 2

Lever length

Lever length is another factor that can be used to progress or regress a yoga pose. In the body, muscles and bones work together to form levers, which allows us to move our bodies and other objects through space. In its simplest form, a lever is a rigid rod that turns about a pivot. The point at which the lever pivots is called a fulcrum. When we move, the bones act as lever arms, the joints act as pivots, and the muscles create a force output to move loads through space. These loads could include one's own body or an external object. The point at which one body part is fixed and another body part is moving is the fulcrum.

Before I delve into how the concept of levers can be applied to yoga poses, I want to mention that this is an overly simplified explanation of one aspect of biomechanics. Human movement is far more complicated than individual joints working independently of one another. It used to be theorized that the skeleton was a collection of bones stacked upon one another connected to individual muscles, which contracted to move us through space. Newer models of movement suggest that the skeleton and muscles are suspended within the soft tissue. When human movement is viewed through these models, every part of the body is an integrated and functional unit. This idea is sometimes referred to as tensegrity, a term coined by Richard Buckminster Fuller, a twentieth-century inventor. Dr Stephen Levin has since expanded on this idea to develop a model of human movement he calls biotensegrity, which applies the principles of tensegrity to biological structures, such as muscles, bones, fascia, ligaments, and tendons. These models emphasize the complexity of movement that occurs in places like joints; however, despite being simplistic, thinking of joints as levers remains beneficial when progressing and regressing yoga poses for your students.

The length of a lever can influence the difficulty of a pose: increasing a lever length will increase the challenge of a pose, and decreasing a lever length will decrease the challenge. A lever length is increased when weight is moved farther away from the fulcrum and is decreased when weight is moved closer. Therefore, poses are progressed by increasing the lever length and regressed by decreasing the lever length.

A simple way to regress a pose is to decrease the lever length by bending a knee or an elbow. Conversely, you could progress a pose by extending a knee or elbow to increase the lever length. To conceptualize this, consider the pose Urdhva Prasarita Padasana or Upward Extended Foot Pose, which is performed by lying supine with legs extended towards the ceiling and lowering and lifting both legs while keeping the pelvis stable. In this pose, the fulcrum is the hip joint, because the pelvis is stable and the femurs are moving. To regress this pose, you could bend both knees to decrease the lever length.

Movement experience for changing the lever length

Jathara Parivartanasana with knees bent: Lie on your back with your legs in tabletop position. Bring your arms out to the sides and press them into the floor.

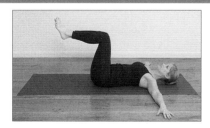

Jathara Parivartanasana with knees bent starting position

Keep your left shoulder blade in contact with the ground as you inhale and take your legs to the right. Exhale to bring your legs back to center. Repeat on the second side. Continue to move your legs to the right and left, and notice the strength required to perform this exercise.

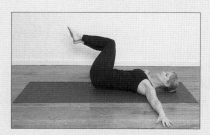

Jathara Parivartanasana with knee sway

Jathara Parivartanasana with knees extended: Lie on your back with your knees extended towards the ceiling, so you have about 90 degrees of hip flexion.

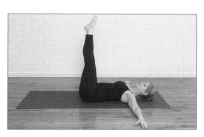

Jathara Parivartanasana with knees extended starting position

Inhale and take your legs to the right, while keeping your left shoulder blade in contact with the floor. Exhale to bring your legs back to center. Repeat on the second side. Continue to move your legs side to side and notice the increased oblique and inner thigh strength required to perform this movement.

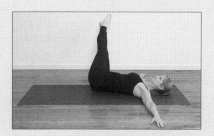

Jathara Parivartanasana with knees extended and swaying to the side

Can you sense how it is more challenging to practice this exercise with your knees extended? This is because there is a longer lever length, which increases the load. Consider how you can apply this concept of lever length to other exercises, so you can regress or progress movements to better meet the needs of yourself and your students.

Chapter 2

Range of motion

Exercises can also be progressed or regressed by adjusting the range of motion, defined as the distance and direction in which a joint can move. Each joint has a normal range of motion that is expressed in degrees, although what is considered normal will depend on the individual. The level of challenge or progression of a pose can be increased by increasing the range of motion, and decreased by decreasing the range of motion. A caveat to this is that people who are hypermobile and able to create large ranges of motion through their joints without muscular control may find practicing an exercise in a smaller range of motion with muscular control more challenging.

One example of this would be Tree Pose. For a student who is not hypermobile, placing the foot on the calf of the standing leg is less challenging than placing the foot on the thigh of the standing leg, because it requires less range of motion in knee flexion, hip external rotation, and hip abduction. However, a hypermobile student might be able to passively rest their foot on the thigh of their standing leg, while locking out their knee joint and collapsing into the hip of their standing leg. For this individual, it may feel more challenging to place their foot on the calf of their standing leg, while activating the muscles around their knee and hip joints to avoid knee hyperextension and collapsing into the hip. This is also an example of how several factors can be utilized to adjust a pose to better meet the needs of your students. In this situation, you have regressed the pose by reducing the range of motion, so your student can better control where their body is in space. However, you have also progressed the pose by increasing the intrinsic load through greater muscle activation.

Regressing Camel Pose by changing the range of motion

One of my favorite regressions for Camel Pose is a somatic exercise sequence I call "prone crocodile," because it teaches students how to find a more effective and comfortable way of coordinating the movement required for spinal extension. Additionally, the prone crocodile sequence involves small amounts of thoracic rotation, while can help prepare the body for extension. Prone crocodile is also an example of how to regress a pose by reducing the range of motion, because it involves less spinal extension than Camel Pose. Below is an example of how I might teach Camel Pose and the prone crocodile sequence in a class setting.

Check: Camel Pose with thoracic rotation. Come into a kneeling position and place a block on the outside edge of each foot on the highest setting.

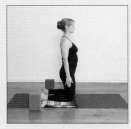

Camel Pose with thoracic rotation starting position

Posteriorly tilt your pelvis and engage your glutes and abdominals. Inhale and reach your left arm up to the sky as you rotate to the right and try to touch the brick near your right foot with your right fingertips.

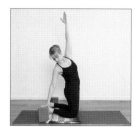

Camel Pose with thoracic rotation

Return to center. Reach your right arm up to the sky. Turn to the left and try to tap the brick that's outside of your left foot with your left fingertips. Repeat this 5 to 10 times. Are you able to find an even amount of extension throughout your spine if you focus more on lifting through your chest and less on sinking into your lower back?

Prone crocodile somatic series

Lie on your belly with your right hand on top of your left hand. Allow your forehead to rest on top of your right hand

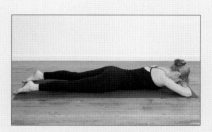

Prone Crocodile starting position

Slowly lift and lower your head off your hands.

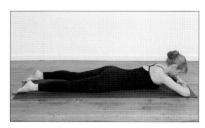

Prone Crocodile with cervical extension

Perform five repetitions and pause in the starting position to notice your breath.

Repeat the process, but this time keep your right hand connected to your forehead, so your head and right arm lift off the floor.

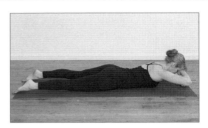

Prone Crocodile with cervical extension and single arm lift

Perform five repetitions. Pause in the starting position and rest as needed. Place your left hand on top of your right and repeat this process on the second side.

Pause in the starting position to rest. Notice your breath as you allow your belly to swell into the floor and your ribs to expand as you inhale. Surrender to gravity as you exhale. Take three to five breaths.

Place your right hand on top of your left and lift your right arm and head as you turn your face and your chest to the right.

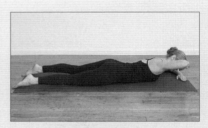

Prone Crocodile with rotation

Slowly lower down. Perform five repetitions. Place your left hand on top of your right and repeat this process on the second side.

Place your right hand over your left one more time. Keeping your forehead connected to your hands, hover both arms and your head off the floor. This should be a small movement. Be mindful to keep the tops of your feet and your pubic bone anchored to the ground. Perform five repetitions.

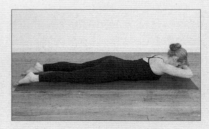

Prone Crocodile with double arm lift

Recheck: Camel Pose with thoracic rotation. Does it feel easier to move through thoracic extension and rotation after practicing the prone salutes in crocodile? How does this compare to your experience of practicing Cobra Pose as a prep for Camel Pose?

Relationship to gravity

Changing the relationship to gravity can also be used to regress or progress a pose. The relationship to gravity is defined as the direction and orientation of the gravitational pull on the body. There are numerous ways to change the relationship to gravity, but some examples would be to practice a pose or movement in prone, supine, side lying, four-point kneeling, seated, or standing. Generally, practicing a pose in a supine or prone position will be less challenging than making the same shape in four-point kneeling or standing.

For example, to alter the relationship to gravity to create a series of regressions for Warrior III, the most regressed version of the pose would be lying supine with one leg reaching up to the ceiling.

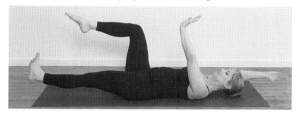

Regress Warrior III by changing the orientation to gravity and practicing the pose in supine.

From there, the pose could be progressed by making the shape in side lying.

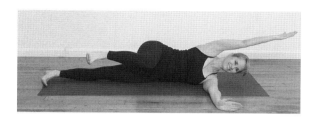

Regress Warrior III by changing the orientation to gravity and practicing the pose in side lying.

The most progressed version would be the full standing version of Warrior III. In this scenario, the supine version is the most regressed or least challenging version of the pose, because more of the body is supported by the floor and fewer joints have to resist gravity. When you are side lying, less of the body is supported by the floor than when you are supine. In standing, you would have to resist the forces of gravity while controlling your body in space without any support from the floor beyond pushing the anchoring foot into the ground.

One caveat to the supine regression of Warrior III is that if an individual has a restriction in their hamstrings, which makes it difficult to maintain hip flexion with knee extension in this position, you might have to further regress the pose by decreasing the range of motion and having the student bend the knee of the leg that is reaching towards the ceiling.

Regressing Eagle Pose by changing the relationship to gravity

Here is an example of how to regress Eagle Pose by changing the orientation to gravity.

Check: Come into Eagle Pose and notice the sensations on the sides of your body. Can you find axial elongation despite having your legs and your arms wrapped around each other? Is it difficult to maintain space between your ribs and your pelvis?

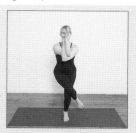

Eagle Pose check

Side-lying Eagle Pose: Lie on your left side. Wrap your left arm on top of your right arm and your right thigh on top of your left thigh. If possible, wrap your right ankle around your left ankle. Lift your head off the floor so it is in line with your spine.

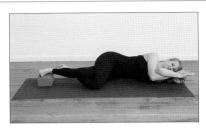

Side-lying Eagle Pose starting position

Press your right knee into the floor to lift your feet and ankles off the ground. Repeat this process on the second side.

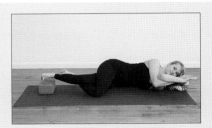

Side-lying Eagle Pose with head and feet elevated

Recheck: Eagle Pose. Has the way that you sense the sides of your body changed? Did the experience of receiving feedback from the floor combined with a change in the orientation to gravity help you discover new areas of your body that you can activate to feel stronger and steadier in Eagle Pose?

Opening or closing the kinetic chain

An open kinetic chain is when the hands or feet are free to move in space. A closed kinetic chain is when one or both hands or feet are fixed against an immobile surface, such as a wall or the ground, and cannot move. Closing the chain or connecting more points to a stable surface will regress a pose. Opening the chain or decreasing the points of contact will progress a pose. To look at this in the context of yoga, let's return to the example of Warrior III. The most progressed or open chain version of this pose would be how it is traditionally performed: with one foot connected to the floor and both hands and the other foot free-floating in space. However, you could regress the pose by closing the kinetic chain and placing one hand on the wall. You could further regress the pose by placing both hands on the wall. The latter has the most points of contact, which is why it is the most closed chain and regressed version of these three examples.

While this deviates from the textbook definition, I often expand the definition of closing a kinetic chain beyond just the hands and feet to include any part of the body that is connected to an immobile surface. This is because the more body parts that are connected to a stable surface, the less challenging a pose will feel. Therefore, a pose can be regressed by closing the kinetic chain and increasing the points of contact to a stable surface, or be progressed by decreasing the points of contact to a stable surface. Some simple examples of this include placing your head against a wall in Plank Pose or making the shape of Warrior III in supine.

If we consider this second example, we can see how orientation to gravity can overlap or be combined with opening and closing the kinetic chain to progress or regress a pose. In the relationship to gravity section, I discussed how Warrior III could be regressed by making the shape in supine, because you don't have to work as hard to resist the forces of gravity to hold the shape as you would in standing. This is also the most regressed version of the pose in terms of closing the kinetic chain (using my expanded definition), because the most body parts are touching the floor, which gives feedback on where you are in space.

It is also possible to partially close a kinetic chain to regress a yoga pose by using props. A partially closed kinetic chain is when one or both hands or feet are able to move but are in physical contact with an object that provides proprioceptive feedback to where a joint is in space. To return to the example of Warrior III, one way to close the kinetic chain would be to place both hands on the wall. However, to partially close the kinetic chain and progress the pose, you could practice Warrior III while holding two cork blocks. The blocks would provide feedback to the shoulders, which could help a student better organize their upper body and balance in Warrior III. Moreover, the blocks are also adding external load. As a result, you are regressing Warrior III from the traditional pose by partially closing the kinetic chain and increasing proprioceptive feedback. On the other hand, you are also progressing the pose by adding external load, which causes the muscles around the shoulder joints to engage more against the increased resistance.

Regressing Side Angle Pose by closing the kinetic chain

Check: Come into Extended Side Angle Pose. Place your bottom elbow on your thigh. Reach your top arm into shoulder flexion along the diagonal.

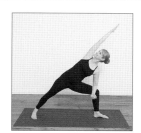

Extended Side Angle Pose check

Extended Side Angle Pose with a block between your knee and the wall: Come into Extended Side Angle Pose with your bottom hand on a block, a block between your knee and the wall, and your top hand pressing into the wall. Can you sense how when you press your top hand into the wall you might be able to find more axial elongation, spinal rotation, and extension? When you press your front knee and your top hand into the wall, is it easier to evenly distribute the weight between your front leg and your back leg?

Recheck: Assume Extended Side Angle Pose without the use of the wall. After experiencing Extended Side Angle Pose with closed kinetic chain feedback for the top hand and the front knee, are you able to create more global tension or a stronger connection from your periphery to your center?

Chapter 2

Unstable surface

Another tool that can be used for progressing a yoga pose is placing part of the body on an unstable surface, such as a bolster, rolled-up yoga mat, or foam yoga block. For example, practicing Tree Pose on a foam yoga block instead of the hard floor, or toe taps while lying lengthwise on a rolled-up yoga mat. The second example also illustrates how factors of progression and regression will cross over: by lying lengthwise on an unstable foam roller or rolled-up yoga mat, you are progressing toe taps by increasing the engagement of the body's stability mechanisms. However, the foam roller or rolled-up mat are also providing proprioceptive feedback on where the pelvis, rib cage, and spine are in space, which partially closes the kinetic chain and could be considered a regression for a student who has difficulty feeling where their rib cage and pelvis are relative to one another.

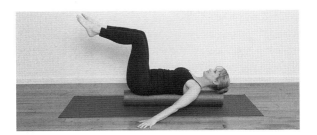

Progress toe taps by introducing an unstable surface starting position

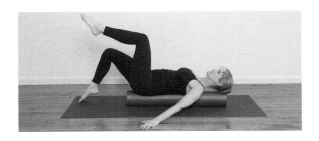

Toe taps on an unstable surface

Exploring Dancer Pose using an unstable surface

Check: Come into Dancer Pose. Notice the connection of the ball of your foot and your heel on the floor. Can you sense a lift in the inner arch of your foot?

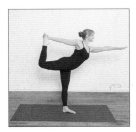

Dancer Pose check

Dancer Pose with foam blocks: Place two foam blocks on the floor horizontally with a two-to-three-inch space in between them. Stand on the blocks with the balls of your feet on the front block, your heel bones on the back block, and the arches of your feet in between the two blocks. Come into Dancer Pose while standing on the blocks. Repeat on the second side. Does the instability and squishy texture of the block create any natural wobbling or perturbation that's more intense than when you practice this pose without the blocks?

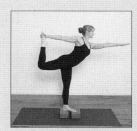

Dancer Pose on foam blocks

Recheck: Resume Dancer Pose on the floor. After practicing this pose on the blocks, is it easier to find your balance in the traditional version of the pose?

Sensory deprivation

Another factor to consider when progressing or regressing a pose is sensory deprivation, which is reducing visual feedback to challenge balance, coordination, and proprioception. An example of using sensory deprivation to progress a pose includes partially or fully closing the eyes: this can be especially challenging for a pose that requires balance such as Tree Pose. However, sensory deprivation can go beyond simply closing the eyes. For instance, if you are accustomed to having mirrors as a reference, you can practice the same poses facing away from the mirrors as a means of progression.

Frequency/volume/duration

The final factors to consider in progression and regression are frequency, volume, and duration. From an exercise science perspective, frequency is the number of training sessions per week. Volume is defined as the amount of work done, such as the number of sets and repetitions. A repetition is the number of times a pose or exercise is practiced. A set is the number of cycles of repetitions that are practiced. Duration

is the length of time spent completing a single bout of exercise. To put this into the context of yoga, frequency would be the number of yoga classes someone took in a week, volume would be the poses that were practiced in each class, and duration would be the length of the individual classes. As a result, when considering progression and regression, these factors apply to both individual poses and one's overall practice. Increasing frequency, volume, or duration will all progress a pose or practice. Decreasing these factors will all regress a pose or practice.

Some examples of using these factors to regress a yoga practice would be to decrease the number of weekly yoga sessions or to practice yoga for an hour instead of an hour and a half. You could also regress an individual pose by holding it for a shorter period or practicing fewer repetitions. Conversely, increasing any of these factors would progress the pose. These factors can also be helpful to consider for injury mitigation. Reducing the frequency, volume, or duration of certain poses or a yoga practice can increase the amount of recovery time between sessions, which can reduce the occurrences of a repetitive stress injury.

Applying the factors of progression and regression to Bird Dog

One regression for Warrior III is Bird Dog, which is also a preparatory exercise that is often used to address cross-body coordination and whole-body stability. Bird Dog can be considered a regression for Warrior III, because it is the same shape as Warrior III, except the lever length has been shortened on the standing leg and the kinetic chain has been closed by placing one hand on the ground, while keeping the other shoulder in flexion. As discussed, the factors of progression and regression can be applied to any yoga pose or exercise. In the following section, I will use Bird Dog to demonstrate how these factors can be adjusted to make an exercise more accessible or more challenging for your students.

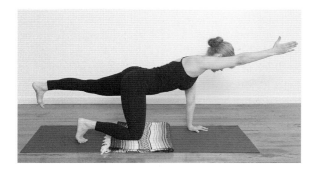

Bird Dog

Bird Dog is already a regression for Warrior III, however, this exercise could be further regressed for a student experiencing wrist discomfort by reducing the lever length of the upper body and placing one or both forearms on blocks. I suggest placing the forearms on blocks instead of the floor to allow students to maintain the same shape as the traditional four-point kneeling position with the torso parallel to the floor.

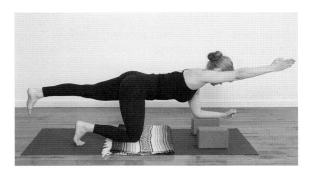

Regress Bird Dog by reducing the lever length of the upper body.

Another challenge that many students face in Bird Dog and other yoga poses is difficulty achieving end range of motion in glenohumeral flexion and external rotation with upward rotation at the scapulothoracic joint. One regression for this would be to reduce the range of motion in the shoulder joint. You could apply this regression to Bird Dog by instructing your students not to lift their arm as high off the ground.

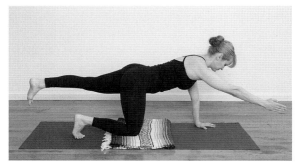

Regress Bird Dog by reducing the lever length of the upper body.

If your student possessed the flexibility to achieve end range of motion in glenohumeral flexion and external rotation with upward rotation at the scapulothoracic joint, but lacked the strength to hold the position, you could also regress the pose by closing the kinetic chain and having them place their lifted hand on a wall. If they lacked the flexibility to hold this position, another option for closing the kinetic chain would be to have them place their hand on the wall with the shoulder in abduction and external rotation instead.

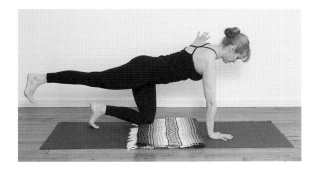

Regress Bird Dog by closing the kinetic chain in the upper body.

Some students may require regressions for Bird Dog that address the lower body. For instance, students may lack range of motion or strength in hip extension. In this situation, one regression might be to reduce

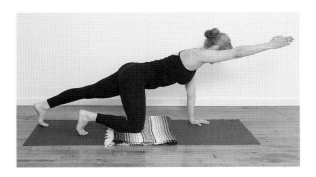

Regress Bird Dog by reducing the range of motion and closing the kinetic chain in the lower body.

the range of motion of the lifted leg by having the student only lift their leg as high as they can without extending the lumbar spine. If the student lacked the strength to do this while maintaining a neutral pelvis, you could further regress the exercise by closing the kinetic chain and having them keep the foot of the extended leg on the ground.

To progress this position while maintaining a closed kinetic chain on the back foot, you could increase the range of motion by having your student place his or her back foot on a wall at hip height. To take this a step further and progress Bird Dog from a closed kinetic chain to a partially closed kinetic chain, you could place a stretchy band around the extended foot and the opposite hand, while floating the back foot off the ground.

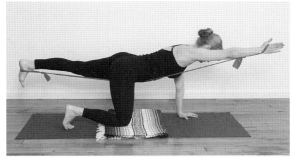

Progress Bird Dog from a closed kinetic chain to a partially closed kinetic chain.

It is also important to note that any of these lower-body regressions can be practiced with or without the upper-body regressions discussed earlier in this section.

The final factors that I have not discussed for Bird Dog are sensory deprivation, unstable surface, relationship to gravity, and frequency, volume, and duration. To progress Bird Dog using sensory deprivation, you could practice the exercise with the eyes partially or fully closed. You could also progress the exercise using an unstable surface by practicing it with one hand or knee on an AIREX pad or foam yoga block. As mentioned earlier in the chapter, you could regress Bird Dog by changing the orientation to gravity by making the shape in supine or side lying. Finally, you could progress the exercise by instructing your students to hold the position for a longer time or by having them practice an increased number of repetitions. Again, these factors can be combined with the regressions and progressions mentioned earlier.

Teacher consideration

Now that you've read about how to apply the factors of progression and regression to Bird Dog, pick another pose and write down how you would apply these factors to this pose when teaching a private session or group class.

Principle 4: Creating an environment of safety

All movement teachers want their students to feel safe and cared for in their classes. This is especially important in yoga, since students can have expectations that classes will improve their mindfulness, reduce stress, and promote well-being. Additionally, many people with a history of trauma or pain, who may be more sensitive to their environment, seek out yoga because it is thought of as gentle and therapeutic. For these reasons, I consider creating an environment of safety foundational when designing my classes.

With the caveat that what can be interpreted as a safe or positive experience is largely subjective, below are my recommendations for creating an environment of safety in your yoga classes.

Recommendations for creating an environment of safety

Begin your class with a pose that is physically accessible for most students and allows them to see what is happening in the room

There is nothing inherently wrong with poses that make it harder to see what is happening around you, such Child's Pose or Downward Facing Dog. However, they may not be an ideal way to start a yoga class, because limiting the ability of the student to initially take in their environment can sometimes induce a startle response. A startle response is an unconscious, defensive response to sudden or threatening stimuli, such as an unexpected noise or sharp movement, which can increase anxiety and fear. A startle response is sometimes preceded by a startle reflex, which is a reflexive reaction from the brain stem to protect vulnerable areas. A startle reflex may manifest as rapid blinking of the eyes or a quick "twitch" that moves through the whole body.

One way to reduce the likelihood of a startle response and help your students feel safe is to begin class with a pose or sequence that allows them to visually orient themselves to the room. This can induce an orienting response, which is when an individual's instinctual response to a change in their surroundings is gradual enough that it does not elicit a startle response. Orienting is beneficial for everyone, but it is particularly important for individuals with a history of trauma or pain. For this reason, I often begin my classes in a seated position or in constructive rest and with somatic exercises. Constructive rest allows students to lie supine in a comfortable position with their eyes open, so they can take notice of the room. During this time, you can invite them to notice where the door is and where the windows are. As you move into somatic movements, you can begin to cue them to turn their eyes and then their heads and notice the objects around them.

In addition to helping students orient to their environment, somatic exercises also prepare the joints for more challenging poses and exercises later in class, which can allow students to comfortably explore larger ranges of motion and assume positions that they might otherwise find uncomfortable. For example, modern postural yoga classes often start with Downward Facing Dog or Child's Pose. As mentioned above, not only can beginning class with a decreased field of vision make orienting difficult, these poses also require end ranges of motion across multiple joints, including shoulder flexion, hip flexion, knee flexion, ankle dorsiflexion, and wrist extension. This can be physically uncomfortable for many individuals if they have not had time to prepare their joints.

Teacher consideration

Consider how you normally start class. Are there any sequences or exercises that you can begin with that might help promote a greater environment of safety for your students? Try creating a sequence to begin class that does not include Child's Pose or Downward Facing Dog. For example, you could experiment with controlled articular rotations, which are defined as movements that occur near or at the end ranges of articular motion with tension and control. You could also try something completely different.

Consider staying at the front of the room for the majority of class

In yoga classes, students are often in vulnerable positions where their field of vision is limited, because they are facing the ground or they are in a relaxed state with their eyes closed. As a result, you may want to consider staying at the front of the room for most of the class, instead of pacing throughout the room.

Standing at the front of the room allows your students to easily locate you at all times, which can help induce an orienting response. It also reduces the risk of you startling a student who does not expect you to walk up to them or past them, because they cannot see you or are in a deeply relaxed state. If you do need to move to another place in the room, you can inform your students where you are moving to, so they have a chance to respond to the change.

Use invitational language and offer alternatives for breathing, positioning, and visual stimulus

Some students who attend yoga classes may have an underlying condition or trauma history that makes a breath pattern, body position, or visual stimulus not appropriate. While teaching a yoga class should not require extensive medical knowledge, offering alternatives can create an environment where students feel safe and empowered to adjust the class to better meet their needs. For example, if you are cueing a specific breath pattern, you can also give students permission to breathe in any way that feels right for them. The same can apply when cueing students to close their eyes. Since closing the eyes might increase anxiety for some individuals, you can invite them to keep their eyes open.

You can also offer options for different body positions and use invitational language when cueing exercises and poses. For example, if you were teaching Warrior II, rather than saying, "Turn your right foot and hip out to a 90-degree angle and your left foot and hip in to a 45-degree angle," consider saying something more general, such as, "Step your feet wide and turn your right foot and right hip out and your left foot and left hip in." From there, you can also give students permission to experiment with their position by asking them to notice how it feels if they turn their back foot and their front foot a little bit more in or out and to pick the position that feels best for them. Using this type of language and providing multiple options will allow your students to learn what positions work best for their body and may prevent them from feeling pressured to perform a pose in a way that might not be right for them, or is physically impossible due to anthropometrics and joint mobility.

Give your students permission to deviate from the positions that you are cueing and demonstrating

Some students will still feel pressured to do exactly what you say even when you provide options and use invitational language. As a result, it is beneficial to give them explicit permission to deviate from what you are cueing and demonstrating. I like to start my class by saying, "You are the boss of your body." By doing this, I am reinforcing that just because I say to do something, it doesn't mean that you need to or that you should.

I actually get excited when I see students doing something different from what I am cueing because I know that they are taking care of themselves. I will also remind them throughout the class that they have the choice to deviate from anything that I am teaching if it doesn't feel right or safe to them for any reason. You can also give people permission to experiment and invite them to make small adjustments.

Be mindful of how you introduce praise

While it can be beneficial to tell your students when they have done something well, you may want to consider avoiding praising individual students during class. Individual praise in a public setting can be problematic for multiple reasons. For individuals from certain cultures and backgrounds, praise can induce feelings of shame. Even if it does not result in shame, praise can also send a signal to students that pleasing their teacher is of greater importance than their experience of the practice. Additionally, praising an individual student can make the students who did not receive praise feel discouraged and can contribute to a sense of needing to perform and compete with the other students. If you do want to offer praise to a student, consider offering it privately after class.

Consider avoiding hands-on assists in a class environment

In Chapter 1, I discussed the potential safety and scope-of-practice issues that hands-on adjustments present. However, I want to include a note about this topic here as well, because it directly relates to creating an environment of safety.

For some students, touch may not be appropriate due to a history of trauma or pain, or an underlying physical condition. Additionally, many students will not expect to be touched, because they assume that yoga will be similar to group fitness classes that they've taken where the teacher stands at the front of the room and demonstrates for the entirety of the class. Also, because many yoga poses involve being in positions where a student's gaze is facing the ground or they are in a relaxed state, they may not notice that a teacher is going to touch them, which could induce a startle reflex. While any unexpected or unwanted touch can be problematic, this issue is compounded in a hands-on assist that takes a student into a deeper range of motion, because it is more invasive than guided touch.

For all these reasons, I recommend teachers avoid hands-on assists when teaching yoga classes. If for some reason, you believe that a gentle or guided touch would be beneficial, be mindful that you receive explicit permission from the student first. If you are unsure, then consider not using touch as a teaching tool in group classes. As a final note, if you are uncomfortable with the idea of using touch for any reason, give yourself permission to never do physical assists or to apply touch when teaching.

How to integrate these principles into your classes

When I was first exposed to the ideas that I share in both this chapter and this book, I was unsure of how to integrate them into my classes, because they felt so different from what I had been taught in my initial yoga training and I didn't want to alienate my students. What I realize now is that it comes down to understanding what kind of teacher you want to be and what you want your students to learn in your classes. In a broader sense, I hope that this book empowers you to feel that you have permission to change how you teach as you learn new things. However, I realize that this isn't always as simple as it sounds. Below are some suggestions for how you can integrate the material in this book into your classes.

First, give yourself time to weave new exercises and ideas into class. I would suggest not changing more than 10 percent of your class at a time. This will give you time to master the new material that you are teaching and will give your students time to learn it. It will also allow your students to acclimate to the shift in your teaching without feeling like they are coming to a completely different class. All of this can help with student retention. One way to do this is to start your class with constructive rest and somatic exercises or sensory feedback techniques in place of the poses with which you normally start. From there, you could teach class in the same way that you normally would. These exercises can feel very relaxing, which makes them feel like yoga, and they can also help prepare the body for challenging poses. As a result, students will typically be open to this type of class introduction (see Chapter 8 for specific exercise ideas).

Another way to integrate new material is to include preparatory exercises that relate to challenging poses that you plan to teach and know will pose a challenge for your students. For example, if you were planning to teach a sequence that included moving through the coronal plane with poses such as Triangle Pose and Half Moon Pose, then you could teach preparatory exercises in side lying earlier in the class to help your students sense the lateral sides of their body through feedback provided from the floor. Alternatively, if you were planning to teach large backbends, such as Wheel Pose or Camel Pose later in the class, you could select preparatory exercises or somatic movements with smaller amounts of spinal extension or thoracic rotation to help prepare the body. Finally, if you were planning to teach a series of poses that required maintaining a neutral spine and neutral pelvis, such as Chair Pose, Warrior III, and Downward Facing Dog, then you could include preparatory exercises that teach that skill in different planes of motion earlier in the class.

There is no universally correct formula for how to format your classes or use this material. However, if you take the time to consider why you are teaching the exercises and poses that you include, then you can give your students a deeper understanding of the purpose of the poses.

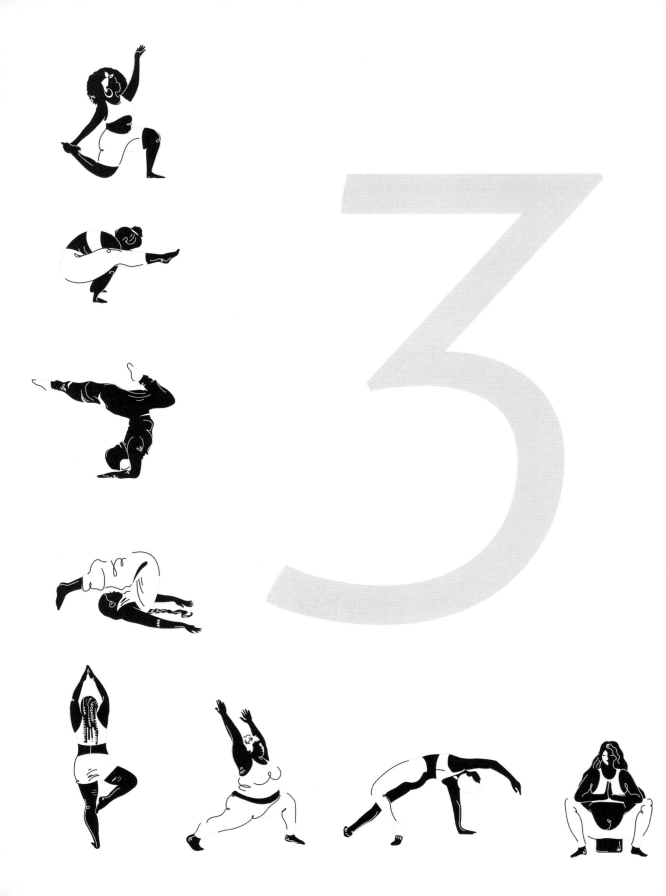

There are three ways of perceiving how we exist in the world, which are known as exteroception, proprioception, and interoception. These forms of perception exist on a spectrum: exteroception and interoception sit at opposite ends, with proprioception in the middle.

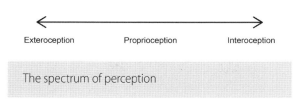

The spectrum of perception

Exteroception is how the body perceives stimulus from the outside world. It takes in this information through sensory nerve endings called exteroceptors. Examples of exteroception include the perception of music and the feeling of the airflow from a ceiling fan on the skin. Interoception is the ability to perceive physical sensations from inside the body that relate to internal organ function, such as hunger, thirst, heart rate, and breath. Proprioception is the subconscious ability to sense where the joints and limbs are in space without visual feedback, through the input of sensory nerve endings located in muscles, tendons, and joints. These sensory nerve endings detect changes in joint angle, muscle tension, pressure, and speed of movement, and send this information to the brain, which tells the body where joints are in space and triggers protective reflexes to slow or stop movements and prevent injury from occurring.

Proprioception versus kinesthesia

In recent years, there has been some debate about the differences between proprioception and kinesthesia. Some researchers limit the definition of proprioception to the ability to assess joint position, while defining kinesthesia as the awareness of joint motion, whereas others consider the terms to be synonymous, or categorize kinesthesia as a subset of proprioception and expand the definition of proprioception to include the ability to sense both joint position and joint movement (Han et al. 2016). In this chapter, I will be using the expanded definition of proprioception, as the ability to sense and integrate both joint position and joint movement.

How proprioception works

There are many different proprioceptors in the human body. However, the primary three related to the musculoskeletal system are the muscle spindle, the Golgi tendon organ, and the Pacinian corpuscle.

The muscle spindle is a stretch receptor found in the belly of skeletal muscles, which senses the amount and speed of stretch being placed on a muscle. When the muscle spindle is stimulated, it may cause the muscle that is being stretched to relax and inhibit the opposing muscle group from contracting. The role of the muscle spindle is to regulate muscle tone and prevent moving too quickly or deeply into a range of motion that could result in injury. When we move into a stretch and sense resistance or an endpoint, that may be the muscle spindle sending a signal to the spinal column indicating that we should not move any deeper into the stretch.

The Golgi tendon organ is a stretch inhibitor located where skeletal muscle and tendons join that senses the amount of tension being placed on a muscle. The Golgi tendon organ is activated when a tendon is stretched: if too much tension is placed on a tendon, then the Golgi tendon organ will inhibit muscle spindle activity, which will cause a muscle to lengthen or relax to prevent injury. An example of Golgi tendon activation in yoga is the ability to move into a deeper range of motion after holding a pose for a sustained period. Holding a low-level stretch can temporarily inhibit the muscle spindle, which reduces muscle tension and allows us to stretch further.

The Pacinian corpuscle is a pressure sensor found in the skin, joints, viscera, and bones, which provides information to the brain about joint position and responds to tactile feedback, such as vibration and mechanical pressure.

Chapter 3

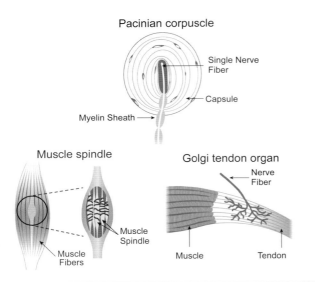

Pacinian corpuscle

Single Nerve Fiber

Capsule

Myelin Sheath

Muscle spindle

Golgi tendon organ

Nerve Fiber

Muscle Spindle

Muscle Fibers

Muscle

Tendon

Proprioception is important because of the role it plays in balance, coordination, and controlling movement. Without proprioception, for example, we wouldn't intuitively be able to sense how high to lift our foot to step onto a curb, or catch ourselves if we trip. In yoga, proprioception helps us sense how deep to go into a pose without overstretching, and where our joints are as we transition between poses or move into end ranges of motion. When proprioception is reduced, we are more susceptible to falling, injury, and pain. This is because impairments in sensing joint position and the natural mechanisms that safeguard against moving too far or too quickly compromise reaction time, making it harder to move with control and precision.

Applying proprioception tests to a yoga class

Tetris click the blocks: Come into tall kneeling holding one cork block in each hand. Reach your arms out to the sides and overhead. Try to connect the blocks by clicking them together in a horizontal fashion.

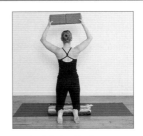

Tetris click the blocks
shoulder flexion

Sweep your arms out to the sides and down by your hips. Try to click the blocks horizontally behind your pelvis. Can you sense if the blocks are matched up?

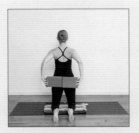

Tetris click the blocks
shoulder extension

Continue this pattern, trying to connect the blocks above your head and behind your pelvis using your sense of proprioception, instead of your sight.

The effects of hypermobility on proprioception

Hypermobility is defined as joint laxity or excessive range of motion at one or several joints. Research has found that individuals with hypermobility syndrome, which is sometimes referred to as generalized joint hypermobility, often have decreased proprioception and are more likely to experience pain (Kirk et al. 1967). An individual's degree of hypermobility is assessed by a screening technique called the Beighton score (Bharat and Lenert 2017).

Hypermobile individuals are potentially more vulnerable to pain and injury in yoga, because modern postural yoga involves holding positions at the end ranges of motion. Hypermobile students are less able to sense where their end ranges of motion are and don't receive the same feedback of muscle engagement or resistance in their joints as non-hypermobile individuals. Consequently, they will have difficulty controlling movements at these ranges of motion and knowing if they have moved too far into a pose. At the same time, hypermobile individuals are more likely to be attracted to yoga than those who are less flexible, because they can easily access the large ranges of motion required for many yoga poses — an ability that is celebrated in social media and mainstream yoga culture.

Joint stability: The ability to control the position and movement at and around a joint by coordinated actions of the tissues and neuromuscular system.

Joint mobility: The ability to actively move a joint through a range of motion. This is different from flexibility, which is how much range of motion you have in a passive position. Mobility is also sometimes defined as the range of motion that you have access to with strength and control.

Generalized joint hypermobility is not uncommon in the general population. It is estimated to be present in up to 57 percent of the population and is more likely to affect women than men. This type of hypermobility is often classified as benign and is different from other hereditary connective tissue disorders, such as Marfan syndrome and Ehlers-Danlos syndrome, which have additional symptoms and health complications. In some cases, generalized joint hypermobility may be a predisposition for high-level athletic performance in activities such as dance, martial arts, and gymnastics, where flexibility offers a competitive advantage. These same individuals may present with lower functional movement capacity, decreased muscle strength, reduced muscular endurance, and increased pain, despite excelling in performance and demonstrating motor control in their sport.

It is theorized that a primary cause of pain for individuals with generalized joint hypermobility is repetitive trauma or repetitive stress injuries due to joint instability stemming from impaired proprioception. Joint instability results in a series of microtraumas to the joint surfaces, which contributes over time to compensatory movement patterns and the overloading of tendons and soft tissue structures around the affected joints. This theory is further supported by evidence that individuals with generalized joint hypermobility have less joint stability and altered neuromuscular activation when compared to individuals who are not hypermobile (Scheper et al. 2015). This can help explain why there appears to be a high prevalence of skilled yoga teachers who identify as hypermobile and develop pain as a result of their yoga practice.

Research suggests exercises emphasizing proprioceptive awareness and joint stability can reduce the negative symptoms associated with joint hypermobility. A study from 2017 found that exercises emphasizing stabilization of the lumbar spine reduced pain and improved stability and muscular endurance in women with generalized joint hypermobility

Chapter 3

(Celenay and Kaya 2017). This suggests it may be beneficial to incorporate exercises emphasizing stability and proprioceptive awareness into our yoga classes, because this type of training can help hypermobile and non-hypermobile students alike. This research is also consistent with the theory that exercises emphasizing proprioceptive awareness can decrease pain and reduce the risk of injury for individuals who have impaired proprioception and pain for reasons other than hypermobility.

Exercises to improve stability and proprioception can be found later in this chapter and in Chapters 5, 6, and 7.

Proprioception and aging

Many factors other than hypermobility can contribute to impaired proprioception, including lack of diverse movement, a sedentary lifestyle, disease, injury, and getting older. Multiple studies have looked at shifts in proprioceptive ability with age. Research indicates that proprioception improves from childhood into adolescence, reaches its height in young adulthood, and gradually deteriorates beyond that point. It is thought that the initial improvement is due to neural development and sensorimotor learning, and the subsequent decline with age is due to a multitude of factors that contribute to changes in the peripheral and central nervous system. Among these changes is a reduction in muscle spindle sensitivity and myelin, which is the insulation found around nerve fibers that allows electrical impulses to transmit quickly (Suetterlin and Sayer 2014). While it has been suggested that a decline in proprioception is a natural part of the aging process, research now supports that a sedentary lifestyle and a lack of diverse movement can influence and accelerate this decline in proprioceptive awareness. Studies have found that active older adults perform better on proprioceptive tasks when compared to their sedentary peers. Examples of proprioceptive tasks include being able to touch the right index finger to the left thumb overhead or opening the hand when the elbow rotates into a predetermined position without watching the movement or using a mirror (Suetterlin and Sayer 2014).

The type of activity also affects how much proprioceptive awareness an individual will have. One study compared the proprioceptive abilities of older adults who swam or ran to older adults who practiced tai chi. It found that while all the active adults performed better than their sedentary counterparts, the adults who practiced tai chi had better proprioceptive awareness than the adults who swam or ran (Li et al. 2008). Studies have also shown that proprioceptive-specific training emphasizing awareness around posture and the spine improved balance and decreased fall risk for women with osteoporosis and kyphosis more than exercise alone (Sinaki et al. 2005; Sinaki and Lynn 2002).

As mentioned in Chapter 1, the number of students over the age of 50 who come to yoga has tripled in recent years (Yoga Journal 2016), and the students most likely to be injured in a yoga class are over the age of 65 (Swain and McGwin 2016). Knowing this, it would make sense that many of the students who come to our classes have limitations in proprioception and as a result may be susceptible to injury. These students would benefit from exercises that emphasize stability and proprioceptive awareness.

The relationship between proprioception and injury

Proprioception can also be compromised as a result of injury. One study examined 20 subjects who had undergone anterior cruciate ligament (ACL) reconstruction surgery. The study found that proprioception was impaired on the leg with the reconstructed ACL when compared to the uninjured side (Courtney et al. 2019). Several studies have found similar results, and it is believed that the reduction in proprioception that occurs after a ligament injury is a result of compromised communication between the sensory organs in the torn ligament and the brain.

Research also suggests that proprioceptive training can mitigate the risk of injury in both athletes and older adults. A study published in the *American Journal of Sports Medicine* looked at the effects of neuromuscular and proprioceptive exercises on reducing the risk of ACL tears in female soccer players. The study found that there was an 88% decrease in the number of ACL tears in the athletes who performed exercises that emphasized joint position and awareness in place of their warm-up when compared to the control group (Mandelbaum et al. 2005). Another study found that postural stability and static and dynamic balance improved in adults over the age of 65 after a 12-week proprioceptive training program (Martinez-Amat et al. 2013), which suggests that this could reduce the risk of falls and increase well-being for aging populations.

Sedentary behavior, persistent pain, and the new model of pain science

Western medicine has segmented healthcare in such a way that we visit a different specialist for each body part or system of the body. For example, for anxiety and depression, we might see a psychologist. For knee pain, we might go to an orthopedist to have the knee evaluated for structural damage. For back pain, we might see a medical provider for an MRI or a chiropractor for an adjustment. Culturally, we view the body through a similar lens. Many people who experience joint pain assume that the problem originates in the area that hurts and will try to alleviate their pain by massaging, stretching, or opting for surgery on that joint. Unfortunately, this approach doesn't seem to work, as evidenced by the fact that America is in the midst of a persistent pain epidemic.

Consider low back pain alone. It is estimated that 80 percent of adults will experience low back pain during their lifetime. In fact, it is one of the leading reasons why people miss work and a main contributor to job-related disability (National Institute of Neurological Disorders and Stroke 2014). However, the problem goes much deeper than low back pain causing missed workdays. According to a study published in the *Journal of Pain*, an estimated 25.3 million adults suffer from daily persistent pain (Nahin 2015). Furthermore, according to the Centers for Disease Control and Prevention (2019), opioids, which are used to treat pain, killed more than 42,000 people in 2016, and more than 40 percent of overdose-related deaths involved a prescription opioid. Given that this myopic approach to addressing pain doesn't seem to be working well for many individuals, or society, it's worth asking what can be done instead.

While it was once believed that pain was indicative of pathology or tissue damage, it's now thought that someone can experience pain long after an injury has healed or without ever incurring structural damage. The most current theory surrounding pain is that it is multifactorial and can be influenced by many things including emotions, physical trauma, lifestyle, and movement habits. Pain is a complex sensory and emotional experience, the purpose of which is to protect us. Although posture, structures and tissues may contribute to the pain experience, they are not linearly related to pain, which is much more complex (Prosko 2019). Nociception is the sensory nervous system's response to potentially harmful or noxious stimuli; it can often lead to acute pain and may sometimes contribute to persistent pain. However, nociception doesn't always lead to pain, and sometimes pain can be experienced without nociception. Some examples of stimuli that may trigger nociception include an extreme change in temperature, an inflammation response within the body, or compressing or stretching a tissue (Prosko 2019).

While there are no such things as pain receptors, we do have specialized free nerve endings called nociceptors, which are located in the skin, muscles, joints, bones, and internal organs, and warn us of potentially harmful stimuli (Moseley 2016). Pain can occur when the nociceptors detect a potentially harmful stimulus and relay warnings to the spinal cord and brain (Dubin and Patapoutian 2010). If these signals arrive at the brain, then they may trigger an output response that causes us to experience pain, as well as changes in breathing, or feelings of fear and anxiety. However, not all of these signals will make it to the brain to create this output. Whether these signals result in pain will depend on whether or not the system detects danger, which will depend on a number of factors, including the nature of the stimulus, the state of the tissues, the state of the nervous systems, hormonal system, immune system, current emotional state, past experiences, and beliefs or expectations around the experience (Prosko 2019).

While the cascade of events described above happens during both acute pain and persistent pain, individuals with persistent pain may have an increased likelihood of experiencing pain even when danger is not present. The problem is that sometimes the nervous system becomes hypervigilant and will send warning signs after the danger has gone or even when danger isn't present (Prosko 2019).

Research has found that the mechanisms underlying persistent pain are different from those of acute pain. In the case of persistent pain, the central nervous system plays a larger role in what causes an individual to experience pain. For instance, individuals with persistent pain conditions, including fibromyalgia, headaches, and temporomandibular joint disorder, will have an increased pain response to normally painful stimuli as well as a pain response to normally non-painful stimuli when compared to individuals without persistent pain. These individuals also have a heightened sensitivity to auditory and visual stimuli. This data suggests that people who experience persistent pain have an issue with heightened sensitivity

of the nervous system rather than tissue damage or pathology in the area of the body where they experience pain (Phillips and Clauw 2011). While the exact physiological process of how this occurs is still being studied, research has found that we have neurotransmitters that can increase or decrease pain transmission in the central nervous system. An increase in the neurotransmitters that heighten nociception or a decrease in neurotransmitters that inhibit nociception could explain why some individuals experience a heightened sense of pain even under low-level stimuli in the absence of tissue damage. This theory has been further supported by research that has found abnormal neurotransmitter levels in individuals with pain disorders, such as fibromyalgia (Phillips and Clauw 2011).

Additionally, when pain persists for a long period of time, there is often a disturbance in body perception around the area that hurts (Lewis and Schweinhardt 2012). Body perception includes proprioceptive awareness, such as the size, weight, and position of one's limbs. However, it also includes the ability to sense temperature, emotions and feelings, and "ownership" of one's limbs. Research has found that individuals with complex regional pain syndrome, which is defined as pain lasting more than six months, had impaired body perception and tactile acuity in areas of pain, and had difficulty accurately sensing size, position, temperature, and pressure in the painful limb when compared to the side that was not in pain (Lewis and Schweinhardt 2012). Body perception can be thought of as the brain's map of the body. Pain or a lack of movement around a joint causes parts of this brain map to get smudged, resulting in a loss of proprioception and the ability to accurately perceive that area. When this happens, sensitivity and pain around that area increases. This is why areas where we have pain often feel "out of joint" or "off" even in the absence of tissue damage (Lehman 2018). This is important to note, because while not all students will identify as having persistent pain, many of them will experience some form of tension or discomfort and will seek yoga to address this. This is borne out in the case of low back pain. An estimated 25 percent of adults in the United States have reported experiencing low back pain for at least one day in the previous three months. To alleviate this pain, the American College of Physicians (2017) recommends yoga as one of the first treatments to try, which tells us that joint discomfort is not uncommon for the average person and that medical professionals are referring their patients to yoga as a way to address it.

Teacher consideration

Think about your students. How many of them have a career that requires a lot of sedentary habits, such as sitting or driving, or standing in one position for long periods? When you teach classes, what are some ways that you can encourage them to include more general movement in their day, which might help them feel better if they have muscular tension? Are there some simple poses or exercises that you can teach in class that they might be able to use outside of the studio?

How language and belief systems may play a role in how we respond to pain

As yoga teachers, it is beyond our scope of practice to diagnose or treat persistent pain. However, because we can improve our students' attentional and interoceptive skills, this may help them manage or control pain. How we cue and teach a pose can impact the likelihood of a student experiencing pain during class. Much of this relates to whether a student believes that a specific pose or movement may be painful or is unsafe. For instance, if a student has a history of experiencing right shoulder pain when they reach their arms overhead, then they may become hyperaware of their right shoulder when practicing overhead movement.

This belief can cause the brain to create an output of pain and fear during any overhead movement, even if there is no danger of tissue damage or injury. This sensitivity can be compounded if the language that is used to teach an exercise or pose reinforces this belief.

Language can potentially act as another input to the system that creates a message of danger. If the words we use create a sense of greater danger or fragility, the system may react by becoming more hypervigilant and protective, even if the student is unaware that this is happening (Prosko 2019). Examples of common cues that may contribute to the experience of pain or anxiety during a pose include: "As you forward fold, bend your knees to protect your spine", or "Engage your core to protect your lower back."

While these types of global claims stem from a well-intentioned desire to keep our students safe, they may not have the intended result. There are many reasons for this. First, these claims are unsubstantiated; there are no data to support that positioning the knee joints or engaging a specific muscle group will prevent injury during low load activities such as yoga. Second, these instructions may result in more fear, less confidence in abilities, less movement options and limit resilience. Additionally, when we listen to the stories from people in pain, they tell us that they often feel guilty or ashamed that they are unable to do what their healthcare provider or therapist is telling them to do. These feelings likely carry over to yoga class: if they believe a specific movement or exercise is supposed to help them, yet doesn't help them and actually makes their pain worse when they try it, then they may feel like they have failed at yet another thing they were told would help their pain.

This can lead to feelings of frustration and a loss of hope. For all these reasons, we want to be thoughtful about the language that we use and ultimately try to bring our students' awareness to themselves to help enhance self-discernment without telling them what or how to feel. Promoting self-awareness and discernment helps with injury prevention and is a key skill to develop when dealing with pain during yoga (Prosko 2019).

Alternative options for cueing to create an environment of safety and exploration

Many yoga teacher trainings have taught us to cue this way, so you may be unsure of what to cue instead. While there is no formula for the right or the best way to cue movement, below are recommendations given by Shelly Prosko, physiotherapist, yoga therapist, and co-author of the textbook *Yoga and Science in Pain Care: Treating the Person in Pain*, on how to update your cueing to cultivate a greater sense of safety and exploration in your classes.

Offer genuine permission

While it is common to say things like "Go at your own pace" or "Use a prop if you need it" in a yoga class, it is important to be aware of how we are presenting these ideas to students. One consideration is making sure all the options that we present in class seem equally valuable. For instance, we can be aware of our tone when we present modifications. Additionally, we can be mindful to avoid statements that make the use of props seem less valuable such as: "If you're unable to do this pose, use a block to make it easier." You may also want to consider avoiding such statements as: "If you're really advanced, then you can..." Finally, be mindful of taking the time to demonstrate different options even if they seem simple, because your students may be unfamiliar with them or may feel empowered to use a prop if a teacher demonstrates how to use it.

Avoid making global claims or directives

Many of us were taught to cue with global claims such as: "As you forward fold, bend your knees to protect your spine", or "Engage your core to protect your lower back." It is also common to hear such statements as: "Back extensions are good for your back", and "Hip openers can release your spine." However, many of these statements are unsubstantiated, may increase the danger detection system to interpret threat or danger, and simply may not be true, because every individual is different.

Rather, you can provide different options for the movements you are teaching. For example, instead of saying, "As you forward fold, bend your knees to protect your spine," you could say, "As you forward fold, bend your knees." From there, suggest different variations for your students to try. For instance, you could ask your students, "How would it feel to bend your knees a little bit more or less?", or "What happens if you turn your feet slightly in or out?" This type of cueing allows your students to have a choice in their experience and to learn what feels best for them in that moment. It also takes away the feeling of needing to perform or the worry that they might be practicing a pose in a way that is wrong or unsafe.

We also want to avoid telling a student when and how to feel things. While it's common for a student to ask, "Where should I feel this?", we want to stay away from telling them that it's right or wrong to have a sensation in a specific place, because it can contribute to a feeling that they have done the movement wrong. Everyone will experience poses differently. Rather, offer ideas to help your student get into a position that might increase awareness of something that you want to address. For example, ask them questions such as, "What happens if you take your right foot back a little bit more?", or "What happens if you lean a little bit to the left?" This type of cueing can direct increased awareness to specific areas without telling students what to feel.

Teach from a place of compassion for yourself and others

Ultimately, the aim in shifting our language is to cultivate safety without inducing fragility or fear. It can be beneficial to reflect on whether the words that you are using come from a place of compassion, confidence, and patience for yourself and your students. You may want to check in with your own internal state, because how you feel will be reflected in your language. Finally, it takes time to adjust how you cue, so when you teach, have compassion and patience for yourself as well as your students.

The relationship between movement and pain

The relationship between movement, alignment, and pain or injury is complicated and still not fully understood. For instance, while movement is recommended to aid recovery from pain and injury, there is conflicting research as to how much the quality or type of movement matters. Additionally, it has been found that too much or too little movement can negatively affect tissue health and increase the propensity for injury. It is also difficult to draw conclusions because the outcome of a treatment depends largely on the individual. Finally, it is still unclear if dysfunctional movement patterns and strength imbalances are the cause or result of pain and injury.

According to recent research (Hodges and Smeets 2015), the suggested relationship between movement and pain can be summarized as follows.

- Movement compensation, which is sometimes referred to as adaptation in motor behavior, can occur in response to pain or injury, when the nervous system senses the threat of pain or injury, or as a secondary response from an additional unknown factor. Examples of a threat of pain or injury include weakness at a joint, too much load placed on a joint, an emotional event, or a sensory experience such as heat or pressure.

- Pain and injury may occur if the body is not well adapted for the loads being placed on the tissues. This includes a large or unexpected load, low-level repetitive loading, a low-level sustained load, or a combination of these loads.

- The relationship between the amount of load, exposure to load, and injury is complicated and depends on the individual.

- In some, but not all, cases, compensatory movement patterns appear to abnormally load the tissues and joints, resulting in pain or injury.

- Some variables that contribute to compensatory movement patterns and which may result in pain include habitually assuming a position, repetitive movement, moving too much or too little in a joint, or too much or too little engagement of a muscle group.

In reading this summary, it becomes clear that the experience of pain and injury is heavily dependent on the individual. However, an important takeaway is that regardless of whether these compensatory movement patterns are the cause or a result of pain or injury, the literature suggests that compensation seems to reinforce the issue and movement re-education can reduce it.

Turning to a real-world example, let's consider someone who has an office job and takes cycling classes as her primary form of exercise. At work, she sits at her desk for most of the day before getting into her car to drive to the gym, where she takes a spin class. The only time that she might not have spent sitting was walking from her car to her desk, or into the gym. As a result, she has trained her body to be well adapted for static spine and hip flexion. Because she sits for most of the day, she seldomly moves through spinal extension, side bending, and rotation. In this scenario, adopting spine and hip flexion won't inherently contribute to joint discomfort or injury. However, many other necessary joint movements are missing, which means some of her joints receive more load while others receive very little. If these movement habits persisted over several years, it might result in weakness in the posterior chain and hip stabilizers. Additionally, she might experience a loss of proprioception around the upper back and pelvis, because she seldom moves through these areas. As discussed, overloading a joint, loss of proprioception, repetitive postures, and issues with muscle firing patterns can contribute to stiffness and pain, so in this scenario, she could develop neck, hip, or low back pain and stiffness.

While this example is hypothetical, it applies to many of our students and explains how an individual might develop pain or discomfort as a result of the structure of the average workday, even if they go to the gym. As yoga teachers, the takeaway is that if we include exercises in our classes that emphasize proprioceptive awareness and load the joints in thoughtful and diverse ways, then we can help our students feel better even if we don't know their full history.

How to choose exercises that better prepare your students for daily life and yoga

As yoga teachers, we do not typically have access to heavier external loads such as dumbbells and weight machines, which are the ideal tools for developing global strength. Instead, our primary tools or loads are bodyweight and small props. As a result, we are best equipped to teach classes that emphasize proprioceptive awareness and help our students build stability and mobility, rather than global strength. In fact, not only do these elements build the foundation for global strength, but they also prepare the body for more advanced asanas, are essential for correcting compensatory movement patterns, and have been found to reduce pain and discomfort for many individuals.

While there are countless exercises and modalities that can be used to foster proprioceptive awareness and in turn stability and mobility, I select exercises and design my classes around three primary methods, which are:

- Sensory feedback techniques: Techniques that involve applying pressure to the connective tissue and muscles to reduce tension and temporarily increase range of motion. Pressure will often be applied with a foam roller or therapy ball.

- Somatic exercises: Gentle movement patterns that shift the central nervous system to create new muscular habits. These exercises are performed consciously with the intention of focusing on the internal experience of the movement, rather than the external appearance or result of the movement.

- Preparatory exercises: Exercises that produce desirable changes in movement strategies, therefore minimizing or eliminating compensation and producing efficient movement patterns.

I use these methods in my classes, because while they deviate from traditional yoga poses, they align well with yoga. For instance, sensory feedback methods and somatic exercises downregulate the nervous system, foster proprioception, reduce joint discomfort, and improve mobility. Preparatory exercises tend to be less relaxing. However, they also foster proprioceptive awareness and emphasize mobility, stability, and in some cases even strength, which can help students practice modern postural yoga poses with less discomfort and create a more sustainable yoga practice. In the following chapters, I discuss each of these methods in detail and include specific exercise sequences that you can incorporate into your own classes.

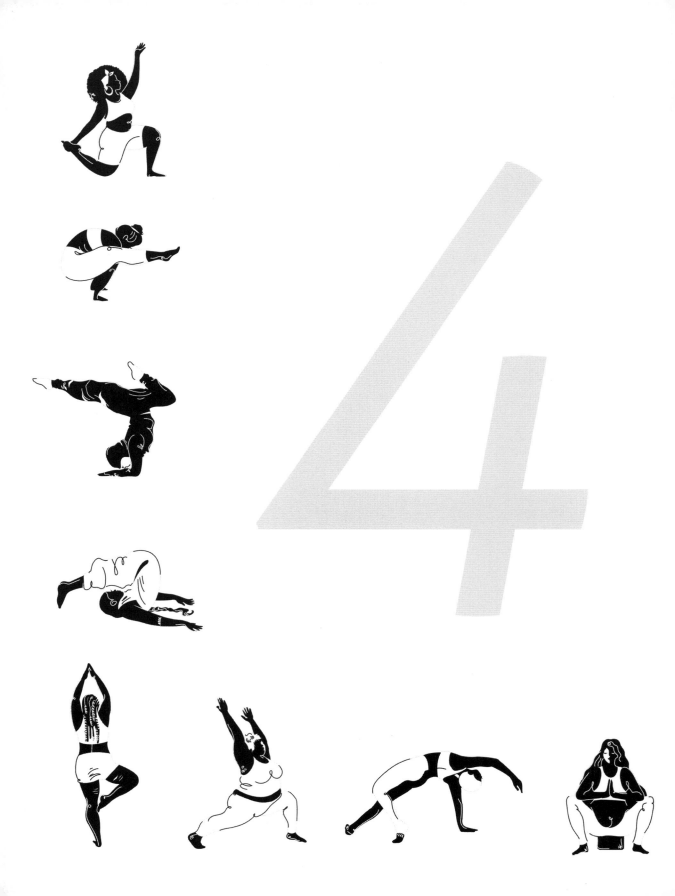

Creating grounding and resilience with interoception

You've probably had the experience of going to a yoga class because it was on your to-do list and because you recognized the need for movement and stress relief. You pry yourself away from that email that needs to be written, get in your car, slog through traffic, frantically look for a parking spot, and dig your yoga mat out of the back seat, before rushing through the studio doors. You enter the studio, unroll your mat, and hopefully remember to turn off your phone. The teacher asks you to lie on your back, close your eyes, and notice your breath. For the first time that day, you surrender to gravity and feel how your body is supported by the ground. All the muscles in your body take a collective sigh of relief and you haven't even done any movement yet. It's like a mini vacation. This is one reason why so many people are drawn to yoga and why they find it life changing. Every class, regardless of style or lineage, encompasses moments like these where we are asked to pause, reflect, and observe. These moments are powerful because they create the space for interoception, which research suggests is why mindfulness practices, such as yoga, are so effective for reducing stress and improving self-regulation.

Interoception and its relationship to mindfulness

Interoception is the ability to accurately sense internal signals from your body, such as hunger, thirst, heart rate, temperature, and breathing patterns. These signals are usually transmitted by unmyelinated sensory nerve endings located in the viscera and connective tissues that project to the insula, which is the part of the brain that helps us identify how we feel about an experience, according to Dr Robert Schleip (2019). How the insula works is still largely unknown, but it has been theorized that it is where visceral states are associated with an emotional experience, and conscious feelings are created (Damasio et al. 2013). It is also believed that interoceptive accuracy is instrumental to how well we manage stress and self-regulate (Critchley and Garfinkel 2017).

You might think the ability to sense interoceptive signals would be automatic; however, culturally, we've been trained to ignore them. For example, when you were in school, you were probably told to sit still and not move until you went to recess. Since children are naturally active, this meant you were taught to ignore your body's signals to move from a young age. For many of us, this carries over into adulthood, where we are funneled into a desk job and continue to tune out these internal signals. The same applies to being unable to differentiate between hunger, thirst, or boredom. From childhood through adulthood, we are bombarded with confusing messaging around food. Meal times revolve around lunch hours and social events without accounting for actual hunger or food preferences.

This tuning out of signals has proven to be problematic, and there's now a known link between impaired interoception and the epidemic of eating disorders, alcoholism, anxiety, and depression. A statistical analysis conducted by the School of Life and Medical Sciences at the University of Hertfordshire found that impaired interoception occurred with a large variety of eating disorders (Jenkinson et al. 2018). Additionally, individuals with major depressive disorder have been found to have impaired interoception, which correlated with abnormal activity in the insula (Eggart et al. 2019). While this information may seem disheartening, clinical studies have suggested that interventions emphasizing interoception are linked with improved emotional well-being, can help treat some disorders, and may be why mindfulness practices are so effective for helping people manage stress.

It is thought that improving interoceptive accuracy through mindfulness practices reduces stress and anxiety because it helps individuals redirect their attention towards what they are sensing, instead of fixating on negative or anxious thoughts (Gibson 2019). One study looked at women in intensive outpatient treatment for substance abuse across three community clinics in the Pacific Northwest. It found that there were significant improvements in self-regulation and mindfulness skills following interoceptive training, which correlated with a reduction in symptoms of depression and addictive feelings. Over time this could suggest better health outcomes (Price et al. 2019).

Chapter 4

Experience interoception through temperature

I normally teach this exploration as part of a sankalpa, which is a positive intention that is happening in the present. If you use sankalpas in your teaching practice, you may want to try integrating this if you have not done so already.

Place your palms together and bring them towards your heart. Start to briskly scrub your palms together to generate heat. Continue this until your hands become warm and start to burn. Close your eyes and place your palms over your eyes, so you can experience the heat of your hands warming your eyes. If you are practicing this as part of a sankalpa, allow the words of your sankalpa to mold their way from the heat of your hands into the back of your eyelids, so your sankalpa sinks into the depths of your brain.

Interoception versus proprioception

Interoception requires slowing down to sense internal signals from the body and noticing how they relate to what we are experiencing emotionally. Unlike proprioception, which is about sensing where our joints are in space, interoception has more to do with how we perceive our internal body. For example, instead of asking, "Which knee is more bent?" you might ask your students, "In which leg are you more at home?" or "Do you feel more energetic tingling in your right arm or your left arm?" after practicing an exercise. You can also invite your students to notice if they are able to sense their heartbeat. These types of questions create mindful curiosity for students and promote better communication between the free nerve endings in the viscera and connective tissue, and the insula (Schleip 2019).

Experience interoceptive awareness of heartbeat through Jnana Mudra

Lie on your back in Savasana or Ardha Savasana or assume a seated or kneeling position if that is more comfortable. Gently connect your index fingers to the tips of your thumbs in Jnana Mudra or the Wisdom Mudra.

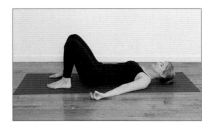

Awareness of heartbeat through Jnana Mudra

Inhale and allow your belly and ribs to expand. On your next exhalation, see if you can lengthen its duration, so it is slightly longer than your inhalation. Complete a few cycles of breathing, noticing the three-dimensional expansion of your rib cage during your inhalation, the natural pause upon the completion of your inhalation, the surrender to gravity during your exhalation, and the natural pause at the end of your exhalation.

Next, draw your awareness to the contact points of your index fingers and the tips of your thumbs. Create a subtle increase of pressure between these contact points. Then, release the pressure. Can you sense a pulsation between your index fingers and the tips of your thumbs? If you can, is there more pulsation in the contact points on your right or your left side? Allow the sensation between your fingertips and thumbs to radiate into your palms. Next, let the pulsation travel from your palms to your forearms, your forearms to your upper arms, your upper arms to your shoulders, across the front of your chest below your collarbones, and finally into the pulsation of your heart inside your chest.

Can you sense how your heart's pace matches the pace of your breath and how they slow down together? Bring your awareness back to the contact points of your index fingers and thumbs. Let the connection be so gentle that it's as if one skin cell of each index finger is contacting one skin cell of each thumb. Observe the pulsation. Very slowly release the contact points of your index fingers and your thumbs. Can you still sense a pulsation even though there is no longer a physical connection?

While enhancing interoceptive awareness can be beneficial for most people, it is especially relevant for anyone with a history of eating disorders, anxiety, or pain, because many of these people report a lack of embodiment or not feeling at home in their body. In many cases, these individuals will have good proprioception, but distorted interoception. For example, research has found that individuals with the eating disorder anorexia nervosa are able to accurately report the degree of lordosis in their lower back or if they have a neutral spine. However, the same individuals reported not feeling at home in parts of their body, difficulty in sensing the heaviness of their legs, and poor temperature regulation, which suggest an impairment in interoception (Schleip 2019).

Another consideration when incorporating interoception into your class is that interoception takes longer for the body to sense and integrate than proprioception. While proprioceptive awareness can happen in a split second, sensing interoception can take one to two seconds. It is thought that this is because interoceptive information is usually transmitted through free nerve endings, which unlike proprioceptors are unmyelinated and have a slower method of neural communication (Schleip 2019).

How to incorporate interoception into a yoga class

There are many elements of yoga that you may already be teaching that promote interoception. For example, Yoga Nidra, meditation practices, and pranayama can help facilitate interoception through the cueing and attention to the breath. In addition, a simple way to incorporate interoception into your classes is to balance movement with moments of stillness. This creates the time for students to become aware of interoceptive signals that they may not notice when they are moving. I often introduce this experience by starting class with a moment of stillness in Ardha Savasana, a pose where you lie on your back with the knees bent and feet flat on the floor.

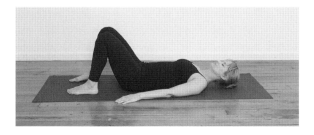

Constructive rest

Once I have invited my students to assume this position, I will prompt them to notice their natural breathing patterns. In some movement practices, this is called constructive rest. From there, I will have them place one hand on their belly and one hand on their lower rib cage, so they can notice if there's movement in these areas while breathing. I will then encourage them to use the inhalation phase to facilitate expansion where they sense a lack of movement.

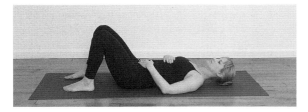

Constructive rest with hands on belly

I might also have them place their hands on the sides or back of their rib cage, so they can sense if they're able to create movement in these places using their breath. Additionally, you can invite your students to notice the rate or the experience of their breath or if they feel at home in their belly and chest.

Beginning class this way is also an effective strategy to help your students become aware of the posterior kinetic chain, which is the back side of the body. Many people have pain around the lumbar spine and shoulder blades, because these are areas of the body that they cannot see. As discussed in Chapter 3, individuals may experience tension or pain in areas where they have impaired proprioception. Unlike in Savasana where the knees are extended and less of the torso is touching the floor, Ardha Savasana allows for more of the back of the body to connect to the floor, which provides additional feedback for the position of the ribs, lumbar spine, and pelvis.

Another option for starting class with a moment of stillness is to have your students practice breathing lying facedown with their foreheads resting on their hands in a pose that is sometimes referred to as Crocodile.

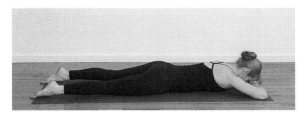

Crocodile Pose

This position mimics the experience of Child's Pose, where students receive tactile feedback on how well their bellies and the front of their ribs move without having to touch those areas with their hands. However, unlike Child's Pose, most people can comfortably assume this position even if they lack mobility in their shoulders, knees, hips, or spine. Additionally, Crocodile Pose facilitates pratyahara for those who have difficulty going inward when they are supine. Pratyahara is defined as the "withdrawal and emancipation of the mind from the domination of the senses and exterior objects" (Iyengar 1979). When we are facedown, we are more likely to close your eyes, which makes it easier to go inward. This means that we are less likely to be distracted by the objects and people around us.

Additional considerations for choosing a pose to pair with a moment of stillness

You might have noticed that it is not uncommon for a modern postural yoga class to also begin with a moment of stillness. However, this moment of stillness is often paired with Child's Pose or a seated posture. While there is nothing inherently wrong with these positions, many people find sitting on the floor uncomfortable or painful. Also, many students have limited mobility in the spine, hips, or knees, which makes Sukhasana and Child's Pose feel inaccessible. It will be difficult to facilitate interoception if students are in an uncomfortable position, because they will find it challenging to remain still and focus on their breath. Instead, they will fidget and be distracted by their discomfort or pain. While props can be used to make seated postures and Child's Pose more comfortable, not all studios have props. Furthermore, many students are resistant to using props, because they feel that props are remedial or only for beginners. This is why I advocate starting class with poses such as Ardha Savasana or Crocodile, where the majority of your students can comfortably assume the position with the minimal use of props.

When I start class in Ardha Savasana or Crocodile, I will often return to the original starting position throughout class and invite students to reflect back to notice if there has been a shift in what they are experiencing physically and emotionally, thus facilitating greater interoceptive awareness. However, these are not the only positions where you can invite your students to sense the changes in their bodies. Any pose can be used to reflect within a moment of stillness. For instance, if you were going to teach a Warrior Pose sequence, you could invite students to notice their breath pattern, as well as the temperature and heaviness of their legs in Mountain Pose prior to practicing the sequence. You could then have them pause in Mountain Pose and notice the change after practicing the sequence on one side. You could return to Mountain Pose a third time to reflect after practicing the sequence on the second side.

When choosing a pose for a moment of stillness, the most important consideration is that the pose is comfortable. For most students, this means assuming a position in supine, side lying, prone, standing, or seated with props as needed, as opposed to a pose such as Warrior III that would require a higher level of strength and balance. Finally, I believe that it is these moments of stillness that distinguish yoga from other mindful movement modalities, because it creates the space for sukha and sthira to promote the balance of effort and ease.

Teacher consideration

Consider the poses and exercises that you often teach. Might one of them be appropriate as a moment of stillness during class, because they facilitate ease and are comfortable for most people to assume?

Using interoceptive cueing with sensory feedback methods

Below is an example of how you can incorporate interoceptive cueing in the check/recheck of a sensory feedback method sequence that you might teach in class.

Check: Stand with your feet hip-width apart with your arms resting by your sides and your eyes closed, if that feels available to you. Notice your feet. Does one side feel more grounded in or connected to the floor? Draw your awareness up your legs. Do you feel more at home in one leg, or does one side feel heavier or lighter?

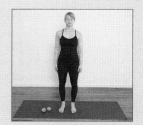

Sensory feedback methods for grounding feet check

Sensory feedback methods for grounding the feet

Place a therapy ball under the ball of your right foot with your heel on the ground. Your left foot should be in a position where you feel like you can balance while you manipulate the ball under your right foot. If you need additional balance assistance, place your hand on a wall.

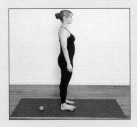

Therapy ball under foot with heel on the ground

Begin to invert and evert your ankle, so you roll the ball across the metatarsal heads of your right foot. Perform five rounds.

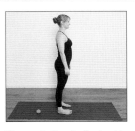

Therapy ball under foot ankle inversion

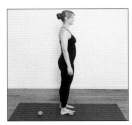

Therapy ball under foot ankle eversion

Place the ball under the arch of your right foot with your heel bone connected to the floor. Flex your toes over the ball. Allow more of your bodyweight to come into your right foot to increase the feeling of pressure or stretch. Be mindful that you maintain tolerable pressure and do not force your range of motion. Perform five rounds.

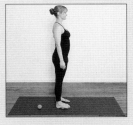

Therapy ball under arch of foot with toes flexed

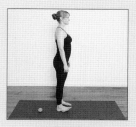

Therapy ball under arch of foot with toes extended

Place the ball underneath the heel of your right foot with the ball of your foot on the ground.

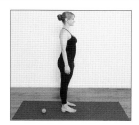

Therapy ball under heel

Swing your heel side to side as you try to squash the ball under your heel.

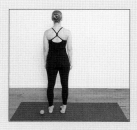

Therapy ball under inner edge of heel

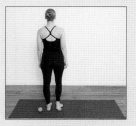

Therapy ball under outer edge of heel

Next, roll the ball from your heel down to the ball of your foot in any areas where it creates a positive sensation. Perform five rounds.

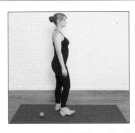

Move therapy ball from heel to toes with ball at heel

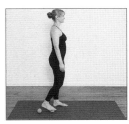

Move therapy ball from heel to toes with ball at toes

Finally, place the ball against a wall, so that it doesn't roll away. Ground the ball of your foot on the floor with your big toe in extension. Lift and lower your heel up to five times to facilitate great toe extension.

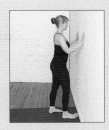

Therapy ball with big toe extension heel down

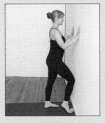

Therapy ball with big toe extension heel lifted

Move your foot along the ball, so your second and third toes are in extension against the ball. Lift and lower your heel up to five times moving through a tolerable range of motion.

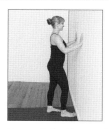

Therapy ball with second and third toes in extension heel down

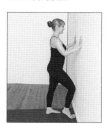

Therapy ball with second and third toes in extension heel lifted

Repeat this process with your fourth and fifth toes in extension against the ball.

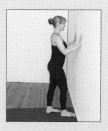

Therapy ball with fourth and fith toes in extension heel down

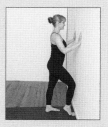

Therapy ball with fourth and fith toes in extension heel lifted

Midpoint recheck: Assume the same position as in the initial check. Notice if there is a greater sense of energy or warmth around your right leg. Notice if your right foot now feels more grounded or if you feel more at home in your right leg.

Perform the ball-rolling sequence outlined above on your left foot.

Final recheck: Return to the initial check position. Sense your right and left feet. Notice if there is a greater sense of energetic tingling, connectedness, or warmth in your feet. Travel your senses up your legs. Notice if you feel more at home or more ease in your legs than you did during the check.

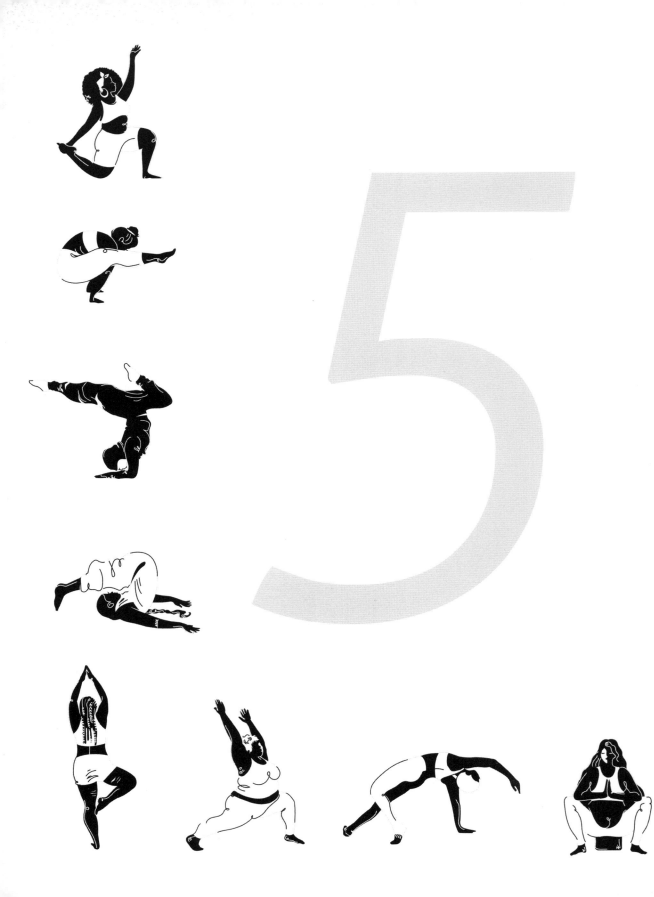

Finding embodiment with sensory feedback methods

When I started taking alignment-based yoga classes early in my career, I was always confused by the shoulder cues. Phrases like "plug your arm bone into your shoulder socket" made me think of electrical outlets, because I didn't know my shoulder had a socket, and if it did, I wasn't sure where it was. I had little understanding of anatomy – I wasn't sure where the bones were, how they were supposed to move, and which muscles were supposed to move them. I found the shoulder blades to be particularly confusing because they were behind me and I couldn't see them. I also had persistent neck and shoulder pain.

The first time I experienced ball rolling was in a workshop. Unlike in a regular yoga class, the instructor showed us where the bones were on a model skeleton, which allowed me to visualize the structures that I couldn't see. She then had us feel where these bones were by rolling on balls. This gave me a chance to feel where my scapulae were in space. By lying on the balls and moving my arms, I could feel how my shoulder blades moved in different directions, while also massaging the muscles that felt sore and tense. When I stood up to do yoga poses, I was better able to follow verbal cues, because I had an awareness around what it felt like to move those body parts. I also had less upper body tension and pain. I later learned that techniques like ball rolling or foam rolling were a way to increase proprioception and decrease the stress response in the body, which was why they worked so well in yoga classes. I call these techniques, which are the subject of this chapter, sensory feedback methods.

Introduction to sensory feedback methods

In Chapter 3, I discussed the specialized sensory receptors in our tissues called proprioceptors, which allow us to sense where our joints are in space. One subset of proprioceptors are mechanoreceptors, which are located in muscles, joints, bones, skin, and connective tissue, and respond to mechanical stimuli, including pressure, touch, stretch, and motion. When mechanoreceptors are stimulated, they initiate a nerve impulse, which is how we detect touch and experience proprioception, or feel where our muscles, bones, and joints are in space.

Additionally, it is thought that stimulating specific mechanoreceptors can help regulate muscle stiffness and temporarily increase available range of motion. It can also affect how our body interprets sensations of pain and movement. One study published in the *International Journal of Therapeutic Massage and Bodywork* found that fascial unwinding or a sense of relaxation happened without the client's conscious control when a therapist applied touch. In its conclusion, the study theorizes that this is due to an involuntary reflex arc that is triggered in the central nervous system in response to mechanical touch (Minasny 2009). While very little research has been done around sensory feedback methods, such as ball or foam rolling, it is thought that this might be why people experience greater flexibility and decreased tension after performing these techniques.

Sensory feedback methods reduce discomfort, induce relaxation, enhance proprioception, and improve range of motion by stimulating the mechanoreceptors through pressure and stretch with the use of tools, such as a foam roller or therapy balls. They can also help students better understand where their joints are and how they move through space, because they give tactile feedback to different areas of the body. While sensory feedback methods are not as specific as hands-on touch, they are a useful modality for yoga teachers to incorporate into classes, because they do not require that you touch your students. This allows you to stay in your scope of practice while mimicking the results of hands-on touch to make yoga poses feel more accessible and comfortable for students.

How to utilize sensory feedback methods in a yoga setting

Many of your students will have too much flexibility in some joints and not enough in others. For example,

Chapter 5

Table 5.1 Sensory receptors

Receptor	Preferred location	Paticular responsiveness
Muscle spindle	Perimysium Endomysium Around epimysial origin of muscular septi	Rapid unexpected elongation
Golgi receptor	Myotendinous junctions Epimysium Joint capsules	Slow elongation of related collagen fibers above a certain strain threshold (may require muscular resistance)
Pacinian corpuscle	Spinal ligaments Inner layer of joint capsules	Rapid changes in local tension and/or compression
Ruffini endings	Outer layer of joint capsules Dura mater Fascia profunda in areas that are frequently exposed to extension	Slow deformation along tangential vectors (shear loading)
Interstitial free nerve endings	Periosteum Subdermal connective tissue (tactile C-fibers) Superficial layers of lumbar fascia Visceral and intramuscular connective tissues	Nociception High threshold mechanoreception Low threshold mechanoreception Polymodal receptivity

Reproduced with permission from Schleip R, 2017. Fascia as a sensory organ. In: Liem T, Tozzi P, Chila A (eds). Fascia in the Osteopathic Field. Edinburgh: Handspring Publishing.

it's common to have excessive flexibility in the lumbar spine and excessive stiffness in the upper part of the thoracic spine. This can be problematic during yoga poses and activities of daily life. You've probably heard of a person who has injured their lower back twisting to get something out of the back seat of their car. This is, in part, because they don't have access to rotation from their thoracic spine, so their rotation came from the lumbar spine instead. The lumbar spine is built to have roughly 5 degrees of rotation in each direction, whereas the thoracic spine should have closer to 30 degrees. So, it makes sense that it wouldn't feel good to rotate primarily from your lumbar spine, which isn't built to perform that action. You can also see how this could present a challenge in a yoga class where the same person might be asked to practice a pose that involves a large rotational movement.

Sensory feedback methods can be used to temporarily increase range of motion in joints that are overly stiff, while increasing awareness around how to stabilize through joints that have too much range of motion. This makes them appropriate for a broad range of students. For instance, hypermobile people are often attracted to yoga because they feel successful when they practice the poses, and stretching feels good in their bodies. They may also come to yoga for stress reduction and because they find stretching relaxing. However, because they may have difficulty sensing their end ranges of motion, these students can experience a greater sense of relaxation when stretching if sensory feedback methods are used.

Hypermobile students will also benefit from the improved proprioception imparted by sensory feedback methods. Applying pressure to areas of hypermobility with balls allows us to feel where our joints are in space. This heightened body awareness can then be applied to practicing yoga, because it gives a greater understanding of which joints are moving and how much we are moving at those joints. Also, if students were previously confused about how a pose was supposed to feel because they lacked proprioception, some traditional yoga cues may start to make more sense in their body.

Conversely, some students may be attracted to yoga because they are stiff and want to improve their flexibility. Many asanas are expressions of end ranges of motion. This can make yoga a frustrating experience for someone who is naturally very stiff, because they are unable to make the shape or match what the teacher is demonstrating, through no fault of their own. Sensory feedback methods are beneficial for these students because they can temporarily increase range of motion, which makes the poses feel more accessible. One study published in the *International Journal of Sports Physical Therapy* studied the effects of self-massaging the calf muscles with a foam roller on ankle mobility. The study found that foam rolling increased ankle range of motion immediately after rolling (Halperin et al. 2014). Additionally, if students feel more successful in class, they are more likely to continue to practice yoga, and over time improve their overall flexibility. By increasing proprioception in joints where many of us are hypermobile, while increasing mobility in areas where we tend to be too stiff, sensory feedback methods can result in better balance and ease of movement throughout the entire system.

How sensory feedback methods can help alleviate discomfort and pain

Sensory feedback methods can also be beneficial for people with pain because they improve proprioception. As discussed in Chapter 3, when we have pain or a lack of movement around a joint, we often experience a loss of proprioception. However, because our nervous system takes the same pathways for proprioception as it does for nociception, or pain, improving proprioception can decrease pain signals (Lehman 2018). Additionally, because sensory feedback methods induce relaxation, they can reduce the stress response in the body, which can potentially have an analgesic effect around areas with heightened sensitivity.

Chapter 5

While there is limited research on the effects of sensory feedback methods on areas of pain or increased sensitivity, there is evidence suggesting that manual therapy can reduce pain signals. According to Carol Davis DPT, an expert in fascia and embodiment, and the author of *Patient Practitioner Interaction: An Experiential Manual for Developing the Art of Patient Care*, "The reason why manual therapy techniques are an effective tool for reducing pain is multifactorial, because the experience of pain is produced by a combination of belief systems, movement history, compensatory patterns, and coping mechanisms. Together these factors create an impact holographically, because what we perceive will manifest within our body" (Davis 2019). Under these circumstances, fostering awareness is a helpful first step, because without awareness there is no choice.

A manual therapist or physical therapist might start with a gentle manual therapy technique that creates a physiological process of pressure and shear to rehydrate the fascia and facilitate awareness and greater ease of movement. However, as yoga teachers, it is beyond our scope of practice to utilize touch in this way, so we can thoughtfully use balls or a foam roller to create a similar effect. Davis recommends using softer tools, because harder tools may apply too much pressure to the lymphatic system. She also advocates moving slowly, to sense the response from the tissue under the roller and adjust the level of slack or pressure to create a greater response within the fascia (Davis 2019).

Using sensory feedback methods to cultivate a sense of safety

Another factor that makes sensory feedback methods powerful is that students can use the techniques on their own bodies, which empowers them to manage their pain without relying on their massage therapist or teacher. Furthermore, for students with pain, the yoga studio can create a safe container for practicing these techniques away from the distractions and stressors that they might experience at home or in a gym. From a psychological perspective, learning these techniques in a group environment can also feel less isolating than practicing them at home, because students can see that everyone benefits from these techniques and that they are taught as a form of wellness, rather than therapy for an ailment. Practicing in a group environment also reduces feelings of anxiety around "doing it wrong," because the teacher is the guide.

For students who don't have physical pain, but struggle with anxiety or attention deficit disorder and find traditional forms of meditation difficult, sensory feedback methods can be a way to meditate without having to be still for long periods. Having a task to focus on and sensations to draw their attention to in a calming environment can create the experience of mindfulness without the requirement of being still in a specific pose or position. Similarly, many students struggle with observing their breath during traditional yoga and meditation practices because they are distracted by trying to position their bodies in the correct alignment. Sensory feedback methods can make it easier to learn a new or more easeful breathing pattern, because students are lying on the floor in a relaxed state. While they might also experience this during Savasana, they are usually checked out and tired by the end of class. Since sensory feedback methods can be introduced early in the class, this allows us to teach breath work when our students are more tuned in to what they are doing and how they feel. Finally, for people who don't feel safe being touched, sensory feedback methods can allow them to experience the benefits of touch and massage while maintaining their sense of control.

Incorporating sensory feedback methods to facilitate embodied learning

We learn primarily through sight, sound, and touch. For many of our students, particularly those who learn kinesthetically, hearing and seeing something might not be enough. Sensory feedback methods offer a way to teach and experience movement through touch without physical contact between teacher and student. It is important to remember that not only do most of us who teach yoga not have a license to touch, but as mentioned in the previous section, some of our students would prefer not to be touched.

Learning movement through touch also gives context for many of the technical cues used in yoga, which might not make sense otherwise. For example, you might be instructed to retract your shoulder blades during Cobra. If you don't understand where your shoulder blades are or what retraction is supposed to feel like, then this cue won't make sense. However, if you were to lie on your back with one ball on either side of your spine between your shoulder blades and squeeze your shoulder blades together, the balls would provide immediate feedback on what it feels like to perform shoulder blade retraction. Then, when you practice Cobra later in the class, you have greater context for what you are supposed to be doing.

Additionally, it is easier to learn and retain information when we receive it in a relaxed state. Technical language can be intimidating and difficult to understand while also trying to execute a yoga pose. Ball rolling helps students embody technical cues, so they can more easily be applied when practicing yoga poses. It also allows them to focus on one thing at a time, rather than having to simultaneously learn a new language and master a yoga pose. This is another reason why I will often teach sensory feedback methods early in my classes and choose sequences around the areas of the body that I want my students to understand, in preparation for more challenging poses that I will teach later in class.

Guidelines and safety precautions for teaching sensory feedback methods

When it comes to sensory feedback methods, there are a lot of theories around application. Below are some general guidelines for how to practice ball rolling or teach it in a class setting.

Do offer a variety of soft and firm tools

For one student, a firmer tool or deeper pressure may feel pleasurable and relaxing. For another, the same tool or amount of pressure can be painful and create a guarding response around the area being rolled, as well as more tension throughout the body. Therefore, it is beneficial to offer a variety of soft and firm balls in your classes. If you are practicing ball rolling at home, you may want to explore using different tools to determine what feels good in your body and gives you the best result.

Exploration of a thoracic mobility sequence using softer versus harder tools

Check: Sphinx with Cat Cow. Lie on your belly with your elbows under your shoulders and your forearms parallel to one another.

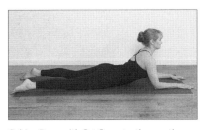

Sphinx Pose with Cat Cow starting position

Chapter 5

Push the floor away and protract your shoulder blades as you drop your chin towards your chest and flex your cervical and thoracic spine. Next, pull your belly in and up as you flex your lumbar spine and posteriorly tilt your pelvis. Your knees should stay on the ground.

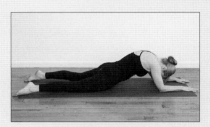

Sphinx Pose with spinal flexion

Reverse directions. Drop your pelvis towards the floor and extend your lumbar and thoracic spine. Finally, extend your cervical spine to bring your gaze towards the ceiling.

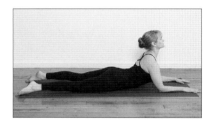

Sphinx Pose with spinal extension

Notice how much spinal extension and flexion you have access to as you practice these movements.

Exploration with a harder tool: Lie on your back with a blanket underneath your head. Place two therapy balls vertically between the medial border of your right scapula and your spine. The top ball will be approximately at T2 or T3, and the bottom ball will be approximately at T4 or T5.

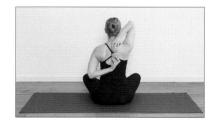

Vertical placement of therapy balls between the medial border of the scapula and the spine with balls between T3 and T5

Wrap your arms around your rib cage as if you are giving yourself a hug. Slowly rotate your thoracic spine to the right and left for six rounds. Notice how the balls will slide into the space between your spine and your shoulder blade.

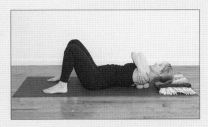

Vertical placement of therapy balls between the medial border of the scapula and the spine

Maintain the vertical orientation of the balls along your spine and move them lower, so the top ball is at approximately T6 or T7 and the bottom ball is at approximately T8 or T9. Wrap your arms around your rib cage and slowly rotate your thoracic spine to the right and left for six rounds.

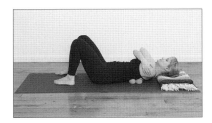

Vertical ball placement between T6 and T9

Maintain the vertical orientation of the balls along your spine and move them lower, so the top ball is at approximately T10 or T11 and the bottom ball is at approximately T11 or T12. Place your hands on your front ribs with your elbows resting on the floor. Take a deep breath in.

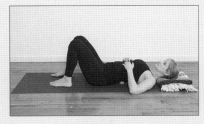

Hands on ribs inhalation

Exhale and draw your ribs in and down as if you are flattening the balls into the floor.

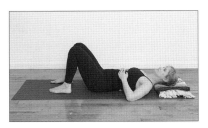

Hands on ribs exhalation

Repeat this sequence on the second side of your spine using the therapy balls.

Exploration with a softer tool: Repeat the sequence outlined above with soft air-filled balls. Do you notice any differences in your experience between using the firm therapy balls and the softer air-filled balls?

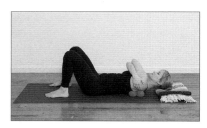

Notice the difference when you use a softer tool

Recheck: Sphinx with Cat Cow. Repeat Sphinx with Cat Cow as described in the original check. Notice if you have more ease or range of motion in spinal extension and flexion.

Don't replace one pain signal with a new pain signal

If you or your student is experiencing pain around a body part, it is unlikely that applying as much force as you can to that area will create lasting relief. While you might feel like something is happening, this type of stimulus is mostly a distraction from the original pain signal. After the ball goes away, the pain will likely return. For some people, the amount of pain might even increase, because applying excessive force can overload the nervous system and create guarding in and around the surrounding areas.

Often the areas where we experience pain are not the root cause of the problem, because as previously discussed, pain is a signal from the nervous system and not well correlated with tissue damage. If you are teaching ball rolling and notice that your students are exhibiting signs of pain or fear, you can recommend using a softer tool, applying less pressure, or moving the ball to a nearby area that isn't as painful to work on.

For some students, even a soft ball can be overwhelming to the nervous system. In this case, they can mimic the movements of ball rolling without the ball. For example, one ball-rolling technique involves placing the ball underneath the shoulder blade and circling the arm for feedback. If this sensation is too intense for your student, then they could lie on their back and circle their arm without the ball, using the feedback from the floor instead. Alternatively, this technique can be practiced against a wall.

Do cultivate a calming environment and encourage exploration of movement and sensation

As discussed earlier in this chapter, promoting a calm environment while ball rolling offers many benefits including greater relaxation, increased learning, and a safe space for experiencing touch for those who have a history of trauma. Additionally, for your students who have pain, ball rolling is a way for them to experience movement and sensation that isn't painful.

Some ways to create a calming environment when teaching or practicing ball rolling include:

- Preparing for ball rolling by first doing breathing techniques either supine or side lying. *This is especially important at the beginning of class*

- Dimming the lights

- Having props available to place under the head when supine or between the knees when side lying for comfort

- Inviting your students to create an intention for their practice or suggesting an intention for those who may not have one in mind

- Reminding your students that they have autonomy and agency, so they have the power to decide if a technique is right for them

Don't roll on one area for too long

The balls are a stimulus for the nervous system and create a stretch in the tissues, so it is possible to overstimulate the nervous system or overstretch the tissues by keeping the ball in one place for too long.

While there isn't a specific rule, I suggest keeping the ball in one spot for a few minutes at a time at most. It is also worth considering the firmness of the ball you are using. The firmer the ball, the less time you need to keep it in one spot. For example, your system would better tolerate an air-filled ball in one place for a longer time than a rubber ball of the same size.

Do perform checks and rechecks when teaching or practicing a ball-rolling sequence

For example, if you were teaching a ball-rolling sequence for the shoulder blades, you might perform a check/recheck by having your students lie on their backs and reach their arms overhead to notice their range of motion. At the end of the sequence, you would cue them to perform the same movement and notice if their range of motion had increased or if their arms felt lighter.

Additional precautions for ball rolling

Stop rolling if you or your student experiences the following:

- Numbness or tingling

- Sharp or shooting pain

- If the sensation is so intense that you hold your breath

- An increase in whole-body tension

- Bruising or excessive soreness immediately after or within 48 hours of rolling

- An intense emotional response

Sensory feedback methods for the forearms and hands

This therapy ball sequence is beneficial for addressing the tensional patterns that develop in the forearms and hands as a result of typing and texting. It can also be used as a tool to improve wrist mobility and help prepare the forearms and wrists for poses such as Downward Facing Dog and Plank Pose.

Check: Place a yoga block between your forearms and bring your wrists into extension, so your hands make a "T."

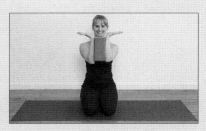

Check wrist extension in forearms "T" position

Notice if your hands look more like a "V."

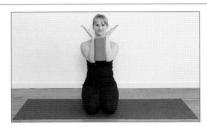

Check wrist extension in forearms "V" position

If this is the case, then you may have limitations in wrist extension and would benefit from greater wrist mobility before loading your wrists in poses such as Downward Facing Dog.

Therapy ball rolling sequence for the forearms and hands

In a standing position, place a blanket or large pillow underneath your right armpit and pin a therapy ball between your right forearm extensors near the elbow and a wall. Lean into the wall until you've achieved a desired amount of pressure. Begin to roll the ball horizontally from side to side. Note, the amount of pressure that you place on your forearm should be tolerable and not induce pain.

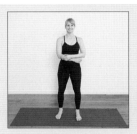

Ball placement when addressing the forearm extensors

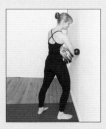

Therapy ball between forearm extensors and wall starting position

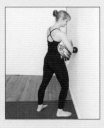

Therapy ball between forearm extensors and wall while rolling the ball

Return the ball to the area near your elbow where you feel the most amount of muscle tissue. Begin to roll the ball vertically along your forearm. Notice how rolling the ball vertically creates a different sensation than rolling the ball horizontally where you are going against the grain of the muscle tissue.

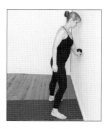

Roll the ball vertically along your forearm starting postion

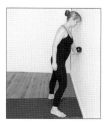

Roll the ball vertically along your forearm second position

Pause on a spot that feels like it would benefit from additional attention. Supinate your forearm, so your palm faces up. Make a fist and curl your knuckles to the inside of your forearm.

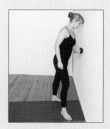

Forearm supination with hand in a fist

Extend your wrist and spread your fingers apart.

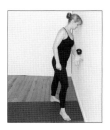

Forearm supination with wrist extension

Alternate between flexing your fingers and wrist and extending your fingers and wrist for six rounds.

Pick a second spot on your forearm extensors that feels like it would benefit from attention. Place the ball on that spot. Slowly pronate and supinate your forearm, so the palm turns up and down.

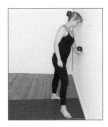

Forearm supination

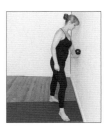

Forearm pronation

Place your forearm across your lower back and pin the ball between the inside of your forearm near your elbow and the wall. Roll the ball horizontally from your elbow to halfway down your forearm. Avoid rolling the ball on the inside of your wrist.

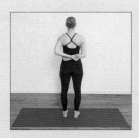

Ball placement when addressing the forearm flexors

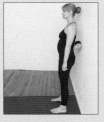

Pin the ball between the inside of your forearm near your elbow and the wall

Pause on a spot and flex and extend your wrist. You can also make circles or wiggle your fingers.

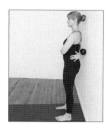

Flex and extend your wrist with the ball pinned between your forearm and the wall

Pin the ball between your thumb and the wall to create passive extension at the thumb.

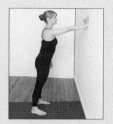

Passive extension at the thumb

Roll the ball underneath your index finger, middle finger, ring finger, and pinky finger, so each finger is taken into extension.

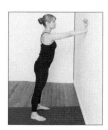

Roll the ball underneath your index finger

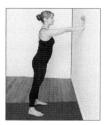

Roll the ball underneath your middle finger

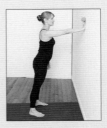

Roll the ball underneath your ring finger

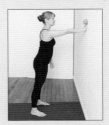

Roll the ball underneath your pinky finger

Perform this action for four rounds.

Pin the ball between the center of your palm and the wall.

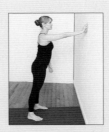

Pin the ball between the center of your palm and the wall

Move your hand side to side, so the ball rolls from the thenar eminence to the hypothenar eminence. If you find an area where you desire more pressure, pause and breathe into that area for two to three cycles of breath.

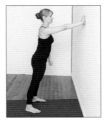

Ball at thenar eminence

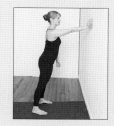

Ball at hypothenar eminence

Repeat the entire sequence on the second side.

Recheck: Place a yoga block between your forearms and bring your wrists into extension, so your hands make a "T." If your hands previously looked more like a "V," are they able to move closer to the "T" position? If this is the case, then you have more available wrist extension than you did in the initial check.

Teacher consideration

Sensory feedback techniques are a beneficial tool for increasing proprioceptive awareness in areas that your students may have difficulty sensing or moving. When considering poses or movements that you are planning to teach in class, is there a specific one that your students struggle with? Could you use sensory feedback methods to enhance awareness of that area of the body, which might help your students be more successful when practicing that movement later in class? For example, if your students often struggle with balance poses and you wanted to emphasize balance, then you could teach a sensory feedback method sequence for the feet prior to introducing single leg standing poses.

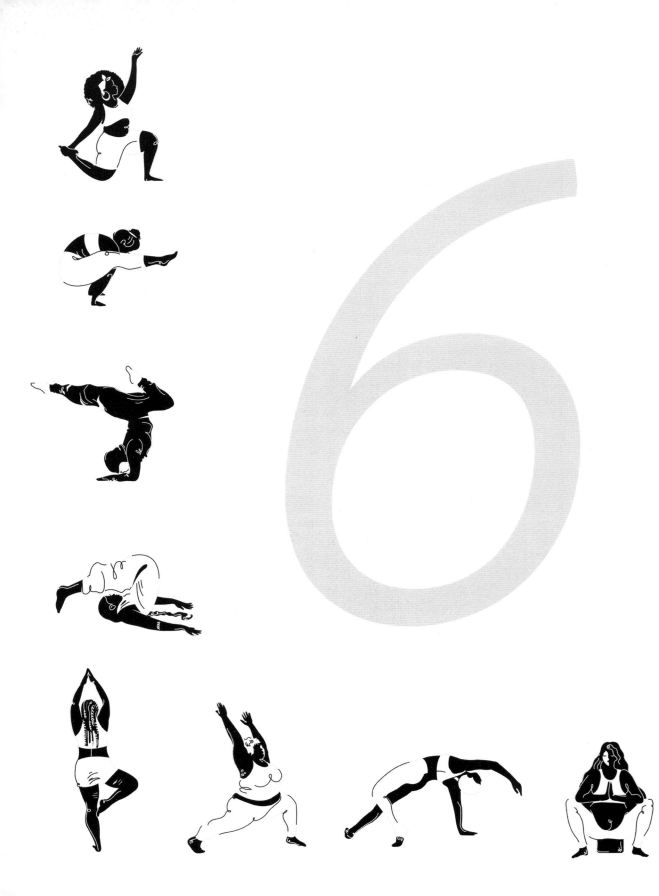

Using somatics to prepare for asana

What is somatic movement, and how is it beneficial?

In the proprioception chapter, I discussed how research has demonstrated that pain does not always originate from the area that hurts or correlate with tissue damage. However, the idea that pain in one area of the body stems from somewhere else and that movement is healing are not new, and have been suggested and explored by many practitioners in the somatic field. Somatics is an area of study within bodywork and movement that takes a holistic approach to working with the individual and emphasizes self-perception and internal experience over aesthetics or alignment. There are several movement systems designed around somatic techniques, including Hanna Somatics, Alexander Technique, and the Feldenkrais Method. However, somatics may also be integrated into bodywork, dance, psychotherapy, and even spiritual practices.

Somatic work is distinguished from other styles of movement in that attention is directed to the internal experience instead of alignment or aesthetics. In a modern postural yoga class, there is often an intention to create a specific alignment within a pose, and to have a sense of having worked hard. This is different from a Feldenkrais class, where working hard would be considered contrary to its ethos, and where movements are slow and subtle, and made with the intention to generate sensory information and attend to that information in a mindful way, according to Todd Hargrove, a Feldenkrais practitioner, Rolfer, and author (2019). This subtle movement coupled with internal awareness is beneficial for enhancing proprioception and creating movement variability, which can reduce tensional patterns and help prepare the body for more challenging yoga poses as well as movements in daily life.

Movement variability can be beneficial for improving proprioception and reducing discomfort in a posture or position, because the part of the body that receives mechanical stress in a movement or posture is constantly shifting, drawing awareness to the sensations that these shifts create. These minor changes in angles can create a sense of relief for someone who has tension in certain positions. While a part of the body that might not always experience work is engaged, a different area has an opportunity to stretch or relax. This also creates a distribution of movement and work throughout the body (Hargrove 2019).

Somatic exercises, such as the ones taught in a Feldenkrais class, create the opportunity for movement variability, because the goal is not to do an exercise with a clearly defined optimal form. Instead, students are invited to practice a basic movement in many different ways. For example, consider spinal rotation. We have 24 different vertebrae that can rotate when we move. If each of those vertebrae participates in a small amount of rotational movement, then rotation will feel easier to do. However, if one vertebra moves a lot and five in a row move very little, then rotation might not feel as good. When practicing a Feldenkrais or somatic exercise, you would be invited to turn your attention to the five vertebrae that were limited in mobility to see if that area is able to participate in rotation, so that all of the joints in the spine can share the load (Hargrove 2019). This is different from how spinal twists are often taught in a modern postural yoga class, where the hands are used to rotate passively into a twist without engaging the muscles around the spine. Also, the emphasis is on moving deeper into a pose rather than noticing which vertebrae are involved in initiating the twist. Additionally, some seated yoga twisting poses, such as Paripurna Matsyendrasana (Complete Lord of the Fishes Pose), emphasize extreme range of motion in the hip joints over spinal mobility, because that is what is required to achieve the aesthetic of the pose.

This increased sense of awareness, control, and mobility can allow students to disperse load and movement more evenly across additional joints instead of

Chapter 6

one or two, making yoga poses more comfortable. This type of non-specific activity can help our students move with more ease both within and outside of their yoga practice, and highlights how somatic movement is different from other mind–body modalities.

How somatics improve mobility and prepare the body for more advanced yoga poses

Many people who come to yoga spend a large part of their day sitting, and consequently move through limited ranges of motion with little awareness. As a result, they may have impaired proprioception and reduced mobility in multiple joints, causing some joints to be underloaded while other joints are overloaded during yoga – particularly if they are taking a modern postural yoga class and moving through sun salutations with a fair amount of speed. This issue applies not just to advanced yoga poses, but also poses that are often classified as restorative, such as Downward Facing Dog and Child's Pose, both of which require large ranges of motion at the glenohumeral, hip, knee, and ankle joints where many students have limited mobility.

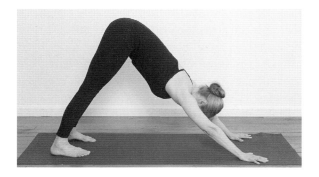

Downward Facing Dog requires end range of motion at the glenohumeral joint in flexion and 90 degrees of flexion at the hip with full knee extension, which is often not available due to restrictions in hamstring length and limitations in ankle dorsiflexion.

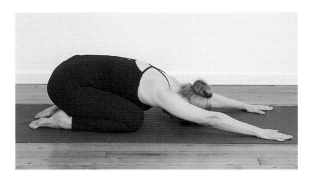

Child's Pose requires access to end range of motion in flexion at the glenohumeral, hip, and knee joints. It also requires end range of motion in ankle plantar flexion.

As discussed in Chapter 3, reduced proprioception, an inability to control the load placed on a joint, too much or too little mobility in a joint, and moving with too much speed or too little control are correlated with increased incidences of pain, injury, and compensatory movement patterns. Somatics can prepare the joints for yoga poses, because they allow students to increase their mobility and gradually progress to larger ranges of motion. This is in part because somatic movements are slow and gentle, allowing a choice of how to move. By moving quickly, the reflexive part of the nervous system is engaged, and there is not enough time to choose or differentiate where movement comes from. While this reflexive ability is essential for moving in daily life and many athletic activities, it can be problematic if relied upon when practicing a movement that is not well prepared for – not taking time to adjust or control the movement of the joints can result in movement compensation.

When a certain range of motion or pattern of muscular activation has been lost, slowing down and paying attention to where a movement is coming from is particularly helpful. The resulting increase in sensory feedback allows this information to be relayed to the part of the brain that develops new movement patterns, and enables adjustment of stress and load (Hargrove 2019).

This process of slowing down is a basic principle of learning new skills: when learning a new movement pattern, we have to be conscious of what is going on. For example, recall what it was like to learn how to drive a car. The first time you drove, you needed to consider where the turn signal, brake, and the accelerator were. However, with practice, this knowledge became more automatic, because governance of those movements was transferred to the lower or less conscious parts of the nervous system.

The same principle applies to regaining joint mobility and sensory awareness that may have been compromised as a result of sedentary behavior and a lack of movement variability. When we slow down and move in a conscious state, we can be mindful and regain mobility and awareness. Over time, the level of speed, load, and range of motion can be gradually increased, to develop these movement skills for the larger patterns required for yoga poses and movements for daily life (Hargrove 2019). While this process is beneficial for all students, it can be especially helpful for students who are hypermobile and often have impaired proprioception in joints that are hypermobile. The increased sensory feedback and awareness from slow, gentle movements can teach students how to sense and control their ranges of motion, which they can later apply to yoga poses requiring larger ranges of motion.

How somatics can reduce tension or pain

Being in pain for a long time can make movement seem stressful and scary. Somatic exercises are a way to give the body information in a relaxed state, improve proprioception, and reduce pain. While it's true that many types of movement could increase proprioception or decrease pain if applied correctly, somatic

exercises work particularly well because of how they are taught. Pain science tells us that a basic function of pain is to protect the body from what the unconscious parts of the brain consider to be a dangerous situation. The brain might consider moving quickly or with increased effort as inherently dangerous for the muscles and joints, because forces are created that can aggravate an area of heightened sensitivity. However, somatics involve moving slowly and mindfully with reduced force and effort, showing the brain that the movement is safe and reducing the likelihood of a pain response (Hargrove 2019). This can help students with pain achieve positions or ranges of motion that might normally cause them pain.

Another theory of modern pain science is that we perceive pain in accordance with something called the virtual body, or brain mapping. These refer to the parts of the brain that track sensory information from the body to protect us and help us move better. However, sometimes parts of this map can get smudged as a result of inactivity in an area of the body, injury, or pain. This can cause the brain to create pain to warn and protect from perceived danger regardless of whether it exists (Lehman 2018).

This idea that we create pain in accordance with perception, or a virtual body, is similar to an idea developed by Moshe Feldenkrais, the somatic teacher and educator with a background in mechanical engineering and physics who created the Feldenkrais Method (Feldenkrais Guild of North America 2019). Feldenkrais believed that we move and feel in accordance with what he referred to as the self-image, or an unconscious perception of what is happening in the body. He theorized that the brain has an unconscious image of the body that senses how it's moving, what it's doing, and how safe it is (Hargrove 2019). His aim was to create a flexible brain rather than a flexible body, because he believed that a positive movement experience sent a series of unconscious signals to the brain that it was safe to move through diverse ranges of motion and positions. This aligns with the idea that changing the experience of pain is about working with the nervous system to decrease sensitivity, and increase safety by correcting smudged parts of the brain map, as opposed to trying to correct a faulty joint (Lehman 2018).

Additionally, somatic exercises are often performed lying down. This makes it easier to surrender to gravity, which is relaxing and can put the body in a parasympathetic state, which is when rest and recovery happens. This is particularly beneficial in a learning environment, because decreasing stress and anxiety makes it easier to learn. One study published in the *International Journal of Neuroscience* looked at the effects of body position on psychological stress when performing mental tasks. It found that participants were more likely to experience anxiety when standing than when lying down. While it is unknown why this happens, it does suggest that being supine could reduce stress and encourage learning in an educational environment (Lipnicki and Byrne 2008).

Lying on the floor also increases proprioception and helps us to understand where our joints are in space. This is significant because, since we are unable to physically see it, most of us don't have an awareness of the back of the body. Also, the average person rarely lies on a hard surface like the floor – couches and beds tend to be soft and provide less sensory feedback. Lying on a firm surface allows us to feel where our bones are relative to one another, which creates positional awareness. For example, when you watch yourself in a mirror during Mountain Pose, you might notice that one of your shoulders is rotated forward. Despite being able to see it, you can't feel it. However, when you lie on your back on the floor, you can feel how one shoulder blade weights more heavily into the ground. This increase in proprioception can translate into sensing where your joints are relative to one another when you

come to standing and no longer have the feedback of the floor.

In addition to offering feedback from the floor, somatic exercises allow us to experience movement in a way that is slow, gentle, and without judgment. When we practice somatics, we are not trying to stretch or make a specific shape. Rather, the intention is to increase our awareness of how our body moves through space. This can be especially beneficial for students who have persistent pain and often feel guilty or ashamed that they're unable to do what a therapist or teacher is telling them to do.

Inviting exploration of movement and internal awareness can reduce the sense of judgment or failure, because it removes the external pressure to achieve a specific alignment or experience a predetermined sensation of muscle activation or stretch. Let's apply this to an exercise. In group fitness classes, crunches are often cued with the intention of feeling the abdominals contract. When this action is performed as a somatic exercise, you might be cued to draw your attention towards how the weight of your ribs transfers into the floor, instead of how the abdominals engage. For example, as you lift your head, you may be prompted to notice how your ribs or shoulder blades get heavier on the ground. As you lie back down, you may be invited to gently press your head into the floor and feel how the bottom of your ribs get lighter on the floor. While both actions involve lifting and lowering the head, they elicit different results.

In the case of a crunch, we may notice burning in our abdominals and tension in our neck and shoulders. When performed as a somatic exercise, we might notice a decrease in effort and a sense of ease in the upper body. This happens because with somatic exercises, there are no mirrors, demonstrations, or cues about the correct way to perform the movement. This reduces performance anxiety over creating the right shape, and shame over "poor" alignment. With somatic exercises, the goal is to do less, not more. This means that you aren't moving to build muscles or burn calories. Rather, you are experiencing natural human movement, which many of us haven't felt since we were children. For our students who are in pain, somatics can create a feeling of safety to explore movement. This way of moving disrupts the tension patterns that manifest from "over-efforting" exercises or staying locked in one position for too long, and reminds us of how movement can be pleasurable, instead of painful.

Rib curl sequence with somatic cueing

Check: Lift and lower your head from supine with your hands interlaced behind your head. Notice if there is any tension across your neck and shoulders.

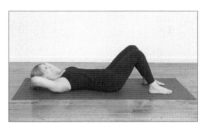

Check starting position

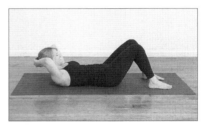

Check spinal flexion

Now, interlace your fingers to cup your skull. Slowly peel your skull and vertebrae sequentially from the floor to lift your head. Lower with control. As you do this, notice the space between your hands and the floor, your head and the floor, and your neck and the floor. Perform up to 10 repetitions.

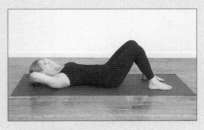

Interlaced fingers at skull

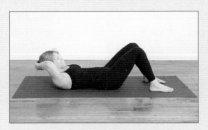

Interlaced fingers at skull with head lifted

Next, repeat the same process, except this time lift your right elbow towards your left knee for up to 10 repetitions. Rest as needed and repeat on the second side. Rest for several focused breaths.

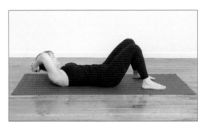

Spinal flexion with rotation to the left

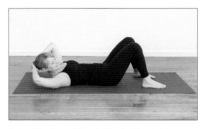

Spinal flexion with rotation to the right

Use your right hand to lift your right knee, keeping the right leg relaxed. Move your right thigh a little to the right. Then, allow your right thigh to drift a little to the left. Try stirring your right thigh in a circle.

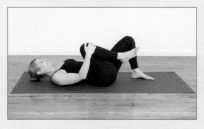

Supported movement of the right thigh

As you do this, see if you can allow your pelvis to remain still and your right foot to dangle towards your right buttock. Also, notice how close you can bring your right knee to your chest, your right armpit, and the midline. Finally, notice how the further you pull your knee towards your torso, the closer that your lower back gets to the floor. Lower your right leg and repeat this exploration on the second side.

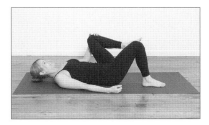

Supported movement of the left thigh

Recheck: Lift and lower your head from supine with your hands interlaced behind your head for five repetitions. Is there less tension or more ease compared to the first time that you practiced this exercise?

Teacher consideration

As yoga teachers, many of us have been taught to cue and practice movement from a place of alignment and aesthetics. As a result, it may be challenging to cue from a place of inquiry. Consider how you might be able to include more questioning or promote more curiosity in your classes to help your students explore movement with less judgment or rigidity.

Incorporating somatics into a yoga class

When we were children, we used the alphabet to make words. Out of words, we learned how to create sentences. Sentences turned into paragraphs and paragraphs turned into stories. You can think of your yoga class like a story, where the alignment cues are the words, the poses are sentences, and sequences are paragraphs. The problem is that most of our students haven't learned the alphabet yet, which is why they struggle with how to execute the actions of the poses. Somatics are a way of teaching students the movement alphabet. By increasing their sensory awareness, they are learning where their joints are and how these joints move through space.

With the exception of movement teachers, the average person probably hasn't thought about anatomy since middle school biology class. Even if they do remember what they were taught, it's likely that they never learned how to apply it to movement, something not usually taught in gym class. Additionally, the majority of people are sedentary for most of the day, so their bodies aren't prepared for asana when they first step on the mat. Somatics give students a way to physically experience anatomy and teach them the key elements that they will need to practice yoga poses.

For this reason, I often include somatic exercises and sequences near the beginning of my classes. As discussed earlier, these movements increase sensory awareness and mobility, which prepares the body for more challenging exercises and poses and may make practicing these movements feel easier and more comfortable. Additionally, if a student has pain or fear around certain positions, somatics may decrease sensitivity and increase a feeling of safety, which may allow them to practice poses and exercises that otherwise feel inaccessible. In Chapter 8, I've provided two somatic sequences in addition to the ones in this chapter. If you choose to include somatic sequences outside of the ones included in this book, I recommend choosing them based on the directions of movement that will be required for the poses that you are planning to include later in class. For example, if I plan to teach a sequence that involves poses with large amounts of spinal extension later in class, then I may include a somatic sequence that emphasizes thoracic rotation and thoracic extension near the beginning of class. This is because thoracic rotation mobilizes the thoracic spine, which makes thoracic extension more accessible. Additionally, if students understand how to extend from their thoracic spine, then they are less likely to overextend from their lumbar spine when performing backbends in poses including Bow Pose or Wheel Pose.

A final note to consider: I typically use somatic exercises as a part of the warm-up for class and spend 8 to 10 minutes teaching a somatic sequence after which I will spend the majority of the rest of the class teaching preparatory exercises as discussed next in Chapter 7.

Using somatics to improve spinal mobility

Check: Come into a kneeling position with your forearms on the floor. Turn your palms to face up and place your forearms at a diagonal, so your forearms make an open triangle shape. Place the crown of your head on the floor in front of your palms. Try to keep equal weight distributed on to each forearm and your head as you slowly roll forward and back in a vertical line from your hairline to the crown of your head. Do you notice any movement in your spine, hips, or shoulder blades as you perform this movement?

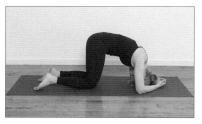

Using somatics to improve spinal mobility check starting position

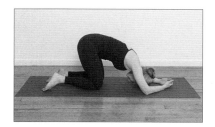

Using somatics to improve spinal mobility check end position

Next, slowly roll your head from side to side as if you were drawing a horizontal line across the crown of your head. Can you do this without using your neck muscles? Do you sense any movement in your spine, rib cage, shoulder blades, or pelvis in response to this exercise? Finally, gently roll your head along various diagonal angles or in any direction that feels good to you.

Sphinx Pose with shoulder blade depression and elevation: Come into Sphinx Pose with your elbows under your shoulders and your forearms parallel to one another. Look forward, so you see the horizon in front of you. Push your forearms into the ground to depress your shoulder blades.

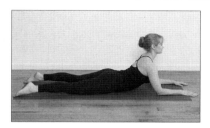

Sphinx Pose with shoulder blade depression

Sink down towards the ground to elevate your shoulder blades. Perform 10 to 15 repetitions.

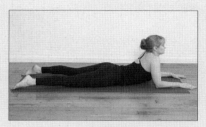

Sphinx Pose with shoulder blade elevation

Sphinx Pose with shoulder blade protraction and retraction: Pause in Sphinx Pose. Begin to protract and retract your shoulder blades. Notice how it feels to slide your shoulders forward as you move your scapulae apart.

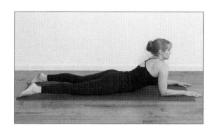

Sphinx Pose with shoulder blade protraction

Then draw your attention to how it feels as you slide your shoulder blades towards one another into retraction.

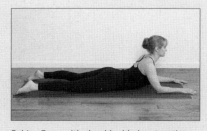

Sphinx Pose with shoulder blade retraction

Perform 10 to 15 repetitions. You can also experiment with allowing your head and cervical spine to move in response to the scapular motion.

Sunbathing position with shoulder blade depression, elevation, protraction, and retraction: Now let's put it all together. Lean back with your elbows under your shoulders and your forearms parallel to one another. Look forward, so you can see the horizon line in front of you. Push into the ground to depress your shoulder blades.

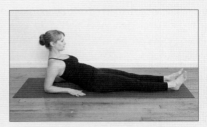

Sunbathing position with shoulder blade depression

Then sink down towards the ground to elevate your shoulder blades.

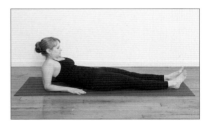

Sunbathing position with shoulder blade elevation

Perform 10 to 15 repetitions. Next, protract and retract your shoulder blades. Notice how it feels to slide your shoulder blades apart in protraction and how it feels as you slide your shoulder blades together in retraction.

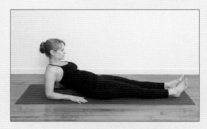

Sunbathing position with shoulder blade protraction

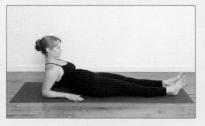

Sunbathing position with shoulder blade retraction

Perform 10 to 15 repetitions, and experiment with allowing your head and cervical spine to move in response to the scapular motion.

Recheck: Come into a kneeling position with your forearms on the floor. Turn your palms face up and place your forearms at a diagonal, so your forearms make an open triangle shape. Place the crown of your head on the floor in front of your palms. Try to keep equal weight distributed on to each forearm and your head as you slowly roll forward and back in a vertical line from your hairline to the crown of your head. Can you notice any movement in your spine, hips, or shoulder blades as you go back and forth? Slowly begin to roll your head from side to side as if you were drawing a horizontal line across the crown of your head. Can you do this without using your neck muscles? Do you notice if this also creates movement in your spine, rib cage, shoulder blades, or pelvis? Finally, gently roll your head along various diagonal angles or in any direction that feels good to you. Has this changed since the beginning of the sequence?

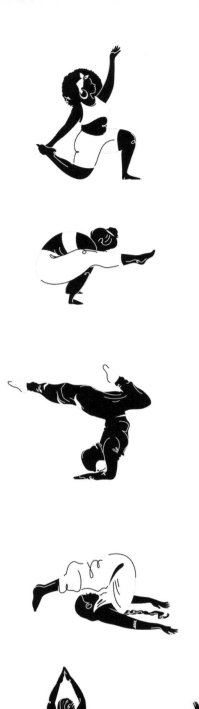

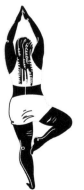

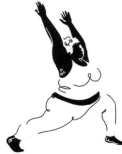

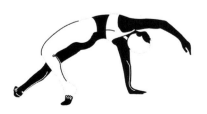

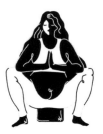

Preparing to load with preparatory exercises

There appears to be a theme among people who experience pain after a long-term dedicated yoga practice. Initially, when they started practicing yoga, it felt therapeutic. The poses made their bodies feel better and even reduced pain. However, a few years into their practice, something shifted. The practice that once made their joints feel better begins to create ongoing wrist, back, or hip pain. Given that this is a common experience among yoga practitioners, it's worth considering why this happens and what we can do about it.

There are a number of reasons why our yoga practice can transition from feeling nurturing to painful, but the issue often begins with why people are drawn to yoga in the first place and how yoga is marketed to the general public. Yoga classes can attract a spectrum of people with differing motivations and ability levels, according to Joanne Elphinston (2019), physiotherapist and author of *The Power and the Grace: A Professional's Guide to Ease and Efficiency in Functional Movement.* At one end of the scale are the very flexible, often hypermobile individuals who richly enjoy the ease with which they can achieve large ranges of motion as they move deeply into their poses. At the other end of the scale are those for whom freedom of mobility is a struggle, but who are determined to overcome their stiffness in the hope that increasing their flexibility will reduce their risk of injury and restore more comfortable movement. This can create a scenario where your class is polarized between the hypermobile students who have the flexibility to create large shapes, but often lack strength and balance to control their range of motion, and stiff or hypomobile students who may be strong depending on what they do outside of class, but don't have the range of motion required to comfortably practice the poses (Elphinston 2019). Even if a student has what might be considered normal levels of flexibility, a typical modern postural yoga class may still not be well designed for them if they have a desk job, because they aren't physically prepared for the poses taught in these classes.

In exercise science, there is a concept known as the SAID principle, which stands for Specific Adaptations to Imposed Demands. The SAID principle states that the body will adapt to the exercises, stressors, and physical demands that are imposed on it. In simple terms, it means that the body will adapt to and be more prepared for the movements that are practiced more often, and less adapted and prepared for the movements that are practiced less often. It also means that when a demand or load is placed on a joint that it is not well prepared for, it may result in pain, discomfort, or injury.

To put this into the context of yoga, most poses taught in a modern postural yoga class require:

- Strength at end ranges of motion across multiple joints
- Mobility in multiple joints
- Stability to control joint position during transitions and when holding poses

Conversely, activities of daily life for the average person who has an office job and sits for a large percentage of their day require:

- Minimal strength in small ranges of motion in very few joints
- Minimal mobility in very few joints
- Minimal stability

Taking into consideration this discrepancy, it makes sense that when we transition from sitting for nine hours a day to adopting extreme ranges of motion, it can result in pain during the poses. While the poses themselves aren't dangerous, many of us are not well prepared for the loads being placed on our joints in class. Additionally, people who are coming to yoga nowadays are less prepared than ever before, because the population is becoming progressively more sedentary with the evolution of technology. With this in mind, if the modern yoga teacher wants to create

Chapter 7

a sustainable yoga practice for themselves and their students, then they need to understand progressive loading principles and incorporate them early on as they guide their clients towards safely undertaking a full traditional yoga class (Elphinston 2019).

Load, tissue capacity, and repetitive stress injuries

In order to better prepare our students for yoga, we need to first understand the different types of load and how preparedness to load relates to injury. It helps to know some basic definitions.

Load is defined as the force exerted on the body. There are two types of load, external and internal load.

External, or extrinsic, load involves moving against a force that is outside of the body. Examples of this include lifting a dumbbell, pushing open a door, or pulling against a resistance band.

Internal, or intrinsic, load is an isometric contraction. Yoga poses almost exclusively involve internal load, because they require holding a pose for a sustained period.

Tissue capacity, or preparedness to load, is defined as the load at which a person is able to perform a movement without experiencing pain or injuring the affected tissues.

While we typically think of movement as influencing muscle, nerve, and connective tissue, all the tissues in the body will adapt to the loads placed upon them. Tissue capacity will vary from person to person and will be influenced by how they load their body during exercise and activities of daily life. When joints are loaded beyond their tissue capacity, it can result in injury, regardless of how technically or accurately the pose is cued. If the tissues cannot support the demands of the loads placed upon them, a compensatory movement pattern may emerge, relieving the stress on the struggling structures but potentially amplifying it in other joints and tissues. However, if the load is reduced, then the student can be guided

to discover alternative and more sustainable loading options (Elphinston 2019). While overloading the joints once will not necessarily lead to pain or injury, it can result in tissue breakdown when done repetitively or if the individual is unable to sufficiently adapt or heal between sessions (Elphinston 2019).

A standard yoga class presents additional issues in respect to loading and building tissue tolerance, because there is a lack of movement variability and diverse loading options. Modern postural yoga classes typically involve flowing through a series of postures where the only props available are a yoga block or a strap, and the primary load is the student's own bodyweight or internal load. When only internal load is available, the body will be almost exclusively loaded in the direction of pushing, and there are few opportunities to load the body and build tissue tolerance in the direction of pulling. This creates an imbalance where the body is better adapted in the direction of pushing and not as well adapted in the direction of pulling. When this is combined with a lack of incremental loading during pushing movements, many yoga practitioners are simultaneously underloading some of their tissues, while overloading others on a regular basis, which if done for a sustained period may result in a repetitive stress injury.

Pain in the nerves, muscles, and tendons as a result of repetitive movement or overuse of a joint is often referred to as a repetitive stress injury, or RSI. A common RSI is carpal tunnel syndrome, which many people have experienced after clicking a computer mouse for eight hours a day, five days a week, over several months or years. An RSI can also occur as a result of repetitive movements during activities, including yoga. One example of a yoga pose that may cause students to load the joints of the upper body beyond their tissue capacity and result in pain and repetitive stress injuries is Chaturanga. It is thought that Chaturanga requires placing roughly half of one's bodyweight on the wrists and shoulders. However, most activities of daily life require minimal loading of these joints: the heaviest object that the average person might push is a door or a shopping cart. As a result, many yoga practitioners will not have the strength to lower themselves down or push themselves up off the ground. In addition to lacking the strength, many yoga students will also lack the scapular, trunk, and glenohumeral stability needed to control the movement. Also, because daily life does not require large amounts of wrist extension, they may not have the wrist mobility required to perform Chaturanga, which requires full wrist extension. Finally, unlike in a fitness setting, where the loads are often external and you can choose from a variety of different-sized dumbbells, in Chaturanga the only option for load is part or all of the student's bodyweight, depending on whether they put their knees on the ground.

This lack of loading options combined with insufficient strength, stability, and mobility means that a student will rely on compensatory movement patterns to perform the movement. Doing a single Chaturanga this way may not be problematic. However, this issue is compounded when Chaturanga is practiced with other poses that present similar or greater physical demands on the wrists and shoulders, such as Upward Facing Dog, Downward Facing Dog, and Wild Thing, which is common in a modern postural yoga class. If these poses are executed dozens of times in a class over the course of weeks and years without enough time to adapt and heal, it can result in an RSI in the wrists or shoulders (Elphinston 2019).

Other examples of RSIs that could potentially occur in yoga include:

- Lower back injuries from too many Forward Folds and Upward Facing Dogs.
- Sacroiliac joint pain, hip pain, and hamstring tears from repetitively moving the hip joints in end ranges of motion in standing and seated poses that mostly focus on external rotation, abduction and flexion of the hips.

- Rotator cuff tears from repeatedly moving from Upward Facing Dog to Downward Facing Dog to Chaturanga with a lack of shoulder strength and stability.

How preparatory exercises reduce the instances of repetitive stress injuries and better prepare the body for yoga poses

While repetitively practicing yoga postures may contribute to pain and repetitive stress injuries, these postures are not inherently dangerous, and we do not need to fear practicing them. There are no bad movements, only movements that are performed too frequently or that tissues are not well adapted for. As discussed above, yoga asanas require the preparedness to load multiple joints in end ranges of motion. One way to prepare the body for this level of loading is to first move in smaller ranges of motion with less load and slowly increase the range of motion and load over time.

Additionally, it is helpful to incorporate pulling movements utilizing external load to counterbalance the repetitive pushing movements practiced in traditional asanas. One strategy to achieve this would be to weight train in addition to practicing yoga. However, because many of our students exclusively practice yoga asanas, it can be useful to incorporate exercises that emphasize smaller movements, external loads, and pulling into our classes as well. Since many yoga studios do not have heavier free weights or the machines found in gyms, an alternative way to introduce external loads is to teach exercises using props, such as stretchy bands, cork yoga bricks, and blankets. Like free weights, prop-based exercises provide loading options beyond one's own bodyweight to help students progressively build the strength to practice yoga poses without movement compensation. Additionally, props create opportunities to practice pulling movements, which cannot be done without external load.

I refer to these exercises as preparatory exercises, because they introduce movement variability and

Chapter 7

develop movement patterns with less compensation to help prepare the joints for the loading demands of physical asanas. Finally, props can help improve proprioception for students who may have less body awareness due to hypermobility or lack of movement experience, because it gives their nervous system greater feedback to where their joints are in space and teaches them how to control the transitions between poses. While any exercise that achieves these objectives can be considered a preparatory exercise, you may find inspiration for preparatory exercises by researching physical therapy exercises, pre-Pilates exercises, and mobility and strength drills.

One reason why preparatory exercises are effective is because they strengthen and stabilize individual joints in smaller ranges of motion. Since many yoga asanas require strength across multiple joints at end ranges of motion, preparatory exercises can be thought of as a deconstructed version of a yoga pose. This makes them an excellent tool to help students assess if they are ready to practice yoga asanas. Additionally, preparatory exercises can help our students become more well-rounded movers. For example, many people will be stronger in the anterior part of their shoulder, because yoga poses and daily life emphasize movements in the pushing direction where the arms are performing a task in front of the body. Knowing this, preparatory exercises can be used to address the posterior muscles of the shoulder to promote better balance in the shoulder girdle. As a result, the shoulder girdle will be better prepared to load in multiple directions, which may reduce the risk of pain or a repetitive stress injury to that joint.

Shoulder stabilization in prone

Lie prone with a folded blanket under your forehead and a strap across the back of your skull. Hold on to each side of the strap with your elbows bent.

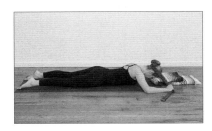

Prone with folded blanket under forehead

Tug the strap apart as you lift your hands and forearms off the ground, so your glenohumeral joint externally rotates.

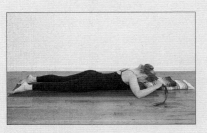

Shoulder stabilization in prone hands and forearms lifted

Perform five rounds. Next, lift your chest as you lift your arms, continuing to tug on the strap.

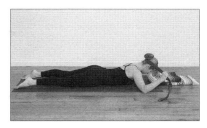

Shoulder stabilization in prone chest lifted

Pause at the top and slowly turn your head right and left for three rounds. Lower with control.

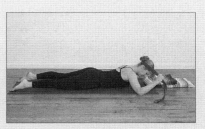

Shoulder stabilization in prone with cervical rotation

The same idea could be applied to other joints as well. For instance, many yoga poses involve passively stretching at the hip joint in external rotation. While this is not a harmful movement for the hip joints, it would be beneficial to use preparatory exercises to strengthen the hip internal and external rotators. This is because strengthening the hip external rotators would help stabilize and support the hip joints in these poses, while strengthening the hip internal rotators would help balance the large amounts of external rotation experienced when practicing yoga.

Experiencing hip external rotation

Lie on your side with your knees bent and your feet in line with your sit bones. Place a looped band around your thighs.

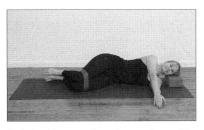

Exploring hip external rotation starting position

Maintaining a neutral spine and neutral pelvis, lift your top knee towards the ceiling. Try to keep your heels together and be mindful that you keep your pelvis stacked throughout the movement.

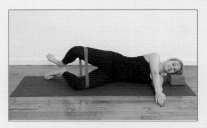

Exploring hip external rotation with hip abduction

Lower your knee with control. Perform up to eight repetitions and repeat on the second side.

Another movement skill that is typically not taught in a traditional yoga class is how to stabilize the spine through core integration. While it is possible to practice poses such as Half Moon or Warrior III without this skill, it often isn't sustainable, because it may result in repeatedly overloading or "hanging" in the lumbar spine or sacroiliac joints, rather than using muscular engagement to control the amount of load going into the joints. Over time, this may cause discomfort in the overloaded joints. In this scenario, preparatory exercises can be used to teach students how to stabilize their spine without the additional challenge of balance and holding a large range of motion. The preparatory exercise regresses the pose, so students can experience core integration without movement compensation, and once they have mastered the regression, then they can apply the skill to a progressed version of the preparatory exercise, which in this example would be the traditional yoga poses.

Core integration with Beast Pose

Come into a four-point kneeling position with a looped band around your thighs. Hover your knees off the ground with a neutral pelvis and spine.

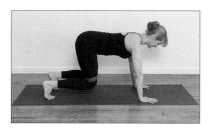

Beast Pose starting position

Step your left foot and right hand forward at the same time while maintaining a neutral pelvis and spine.

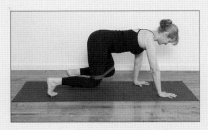

Beast Pose left foot and right hand stepped forward

Repeat on the second side. Perform four to eight steps forward and then repeat going backwards.

Preparatory exercises can be used as an assessment during class to help students identify if they have the strength and stability to control specific joints at the end ranges of motion required for asanas and understand why certain postures may create discomfort or pain. Additionally, if you are a yoga teacher, then you can use preparatory exercises in the form of assessments to help your students understand why you are deviating from the traditional class format that they may be accustomed to. If your students are able to feel the changes in their body during class and experience less pain or difficulty in a pose that they struggle with, then they may be more likely to return to your class and might even request more preparatory exercises in the future.

How to choose preparatory exercises for classes

When choosing which preparatory exercises to teach, it can be helpful to consider how they relate to a pose that your students struggle with. This will allow you to pick exercises specific to your students' needs and will help your students assess if they are ready to practice the pose in question. When you consider a specific pose, think about why your students might find that position challenging. As discussed in the beginning of the chapter, some students will lack the passive range of motion or flexibility in one or several joints to perform the pose. Often these students will experience discomfort when they practice the pose, because they are trying to force a range of motion in their joints that they don't have access to. However, they won't understand that the discomfort is due to a lack of flexibility and will try to push through it, which in turn increases the discomfort.

In other instances, a student will have the flexibility to practice the pose, but may lack the strength and control to hold the position. This causes them to collapse into their joints and results in discomfort or pain in the overloaded joints. Additionally, while some students may have the strength and control to comfortably practice individual poses, they may lack the strength to transition between poses, which might create pain during the transitions. Finally, some students may be under the impression that the correct way to practice a pose is by going into the deepest range of motion possible. In these cases, they may not realize that they are collapsing into their joints or experience pain in the moment. However, over time this may result in pain because of the repetitive stress placed on the joints.

While individuals may experience discomfort during yoga for different reasons, ultimately if you select exercises that emphasize joint mobility, joint stability, and strength, then all of your students will be better prepared for the movements of traditional asanas.

When choosing which exercises to teach, I follow a simple three-step process:

1. Identify the directions of movement required to practice the pose.

2. Consider the physical demands within each direction of movement and the movement compensations that may occur if students do not have the movement skills to meet these physical demands.

3. Select exercises to help students meet the physical demands of the pose for each direction of movement.

Let's apply this selection process to Downward Facing Dog, a pose that many of our students will struggle with and will often be asked to practice multiple times during a modern postural yoga class.

First, the primary directions of movement are:

- Shoulder flexion

- Wrist extension

- Hip flexion

- Ankle dorsiflexion

Now consider the physical requirements for each of these elements, and the movement compensations or limitations that will help identify if students do not have these skills: in this case, starting with shoulder flexion.

Shoulder flexion occurs when we move our arms from the sides, out in front, and into an overhead position. Many people are limited in shoulder flexion, because the movement is not commonly used in daily life, and is seldom practiced. Even if people regularly do lift their arms overhead, they are unlikely to do so with much external load. However, Downward Facing Dog requires:

- The mobility to bring the arms into full shoulder flexion.

- The strength to support a significant percentage of one's own bodyweight with the arms in full shoulder flexion.

- The stability to control the spine, pelvis, and glenohumeral and scapulothoracic joints.

Now consider what we might see if a student does not have the shoulder mobility required for Downward Facing Dog. For example, a common movement compensation for impaired mobility in shoulder flexion is that the spine appears overly extended or collapsed when holding Downward Facing Dog. This happens because the student has unconsciously hyperextended part of the spine to make up for the range of motion that is unavailable in the glenohumeral joint.

Additional movement compensations that may occur as a result of limitations in shoulder flexion mobility or a lack of shoulder stability and strength include:

- Forward head posture or an anterior translation of the skull when the arms reach overhead.

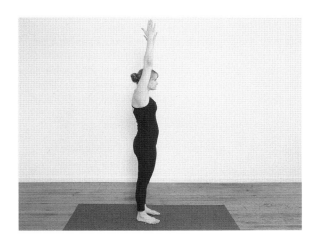

Anterior translation of the skull when arms reach overhead

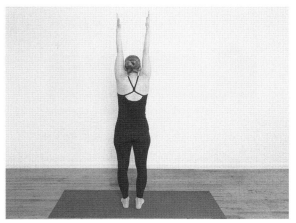

Shoulder elevation and protraction

While these compensations will not always manifest in Downward Facing Dog, I mention them because you may see them when your students are practicing other preparatory exercises or poses during class.

- Elevating and protracting the shoulder blades in place of upward rotation. This will often look like the shoulder blades are "shrugging" up to the ears.

Below is a sequence that I might use to help students prepare their shoulders for Downward Facing Dog.

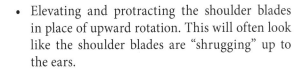

Shoulder flexion for Downward Facing Dog

Supine knees-bent single-arm overhead reach

Lie on your back with your knees bent and your feet flat on the floor. Inhale to expand your belly and ribs three-dimensionally. Exhale to create pressure outwards and brace your core. Externally rotate your right shoulder and supinate your forearm.

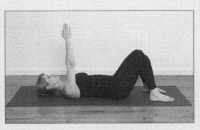

Supine knees-bent single-arm overhead reach starting position

Reach your arm overhead while maintaining a neutral pelvis and spine, pausing before your mid back leaves the floor.

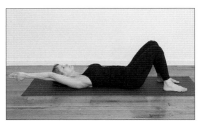

Supine knees-bent single-arm overhead reach ending position

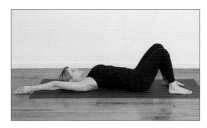

An example of what it looks like when the mid ribs leave the ground. Ideally, they should stay connected to the floor for the entire movement.

Lower your arm with control and repeat on the second side.

Supine knees-bent double-arm overhead reach with strap supinated grip

Lie on your back with your knees bent and your feet flat on the floor. Inhale to expand your belly and ribs three-dimensionally. Exhale to create pressure outwards and brace your core. Hold on to a strap with both hands. Externally rotate your shoulders and supinate your forearms.

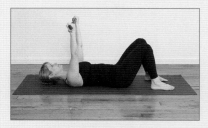

Supine knees-bent double-arm overhead reach with strap supinated grip starting position

Pull the strap apart as you reach both arms overhead while maintaining a neutral pelvis and spine, pausing before your mid back leaves the floor.

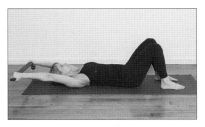

Supine knees-bent double-arm overhead reach with strap supinated grip ending position

Lower your arms with control. Perform five rounds.

Four-point kneeling single-arm overhead reach

Come into a quadruped position.

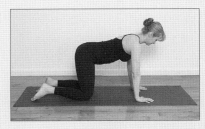

Four-point kneeling single arm overhead reach starting position

Reach your right arm in front of you. Externally rotate your right shoulder and supinate your right forearm so that your right thumb is pointing towards the ceiling. Lift your arm into shoulder flexion while maintaining a neutral pelvis and neutral spine. Notice the upward rotation of your right shoulder blade.

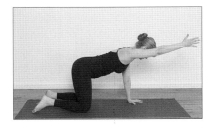

Four-point kneeling single arm overhead reach with shoulder flexion

Lower your right arm with control. Perform five rounds and repeat on the left side.

107

Four-point kneeling single-arm overhead reach holding brick

Place a brick on the right side of your mat. Come into a quadruped position. Reach your right arm in front of you and grasp the brick in your hand.

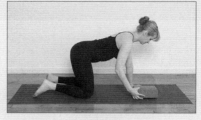

Four-point kneeling single arm overhead reach holding brick starting position

Externally rotate your right shoulder and supinate your right forearm so that your right thumb is pointing towards the ceiling. Lift your arm into shoulder flexion while maintaining a neutral pelvis and neutral spine. Notice how the brick provides external load and changes the experience of the exercise.

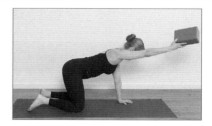

Four-point kneeling single arm overhead reach holding brick with shoulder flexion

Lower your right arm with control. Perform five rounds and repeat on the left side.

Having completed this process for shoulder flexion, the next direction of movement on the list to be addressed is wrist extension.

Wrist extension occurs when the back of the hand is pulled back towards the back of the forearm. As with shoulder flexion, wrist extension is rarely required in daily life, and unlikely to be performed under load. For this reason, many of our students lack wrist mobility and the tissue tolerance to bear weight in wrist extension. As a result, they may experience pain or discomfort in Downward Facing Dog, because the pose requires loading the wrists in extension with a significant amount of one's bodyweight.

Students with limitations in wrist extension may present with one or all of the following movement compensations during Downward Facing Dog:

- Internal rotation at the glenohumeral joint

- Elbows that appear bent or the inability to fully straighten the elbows

- Shoulders that appear to "shrug" into the ears

It is worth noting that the above compensations can also occur if someone is limited in shoulder flexion. However, many of our students will have limitations in both shoulder flexion and wrist extension, so it is beneficial to address both of these areas with preparatory exercises.

Here are some exercises to address wrist extension and help prepare the wrists for loading in positions such as Downward Facing Dog.

Wrist loading for Downward Facing Dog

Check: Prayer palms "V" versus "T." Bring your palms and forearms together in front of you.

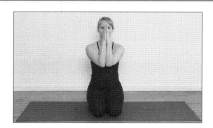

Prayer palms "V" vs. "T" starting position

Extend your wrists to their comfortable end range. Notice how much range of motion you have in wrist extension by observing if your arms and hands look more like the letter "V" or the letter "T".

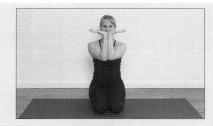

Prayer palms "T"

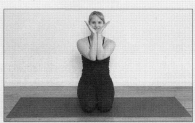

Prayer palms "V"

If your hands look more like the letter "V", then it means that you may have limited mobility in wrist extension, which could contribute to wrist discomfort when you load the wrists in extension during poses such as Downward Facing Dog or Chaturanga.

Four-point kneeling shifting weight in all directions

Come onto your hands and knees with your wrists under your shoulders and your knees under your hips.

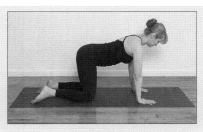

Four-point kneeling shifting weight in all directions starting position

Shift your bodyweight from side to side. Notice how the loading of your bodyweight will shift from your right hand to your left hand.

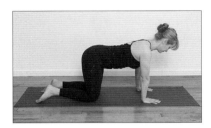

Four-point kneeling weight shift to right

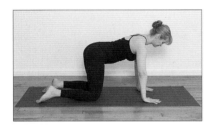

Four-point kneeling weight shift to left

Next, shift your weight forward and back. Notice how the loading of your bodyweight will move from the heels of your hands to your fingertips.

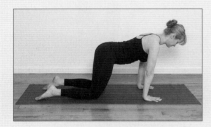

Four-point kneeling weight shift forward

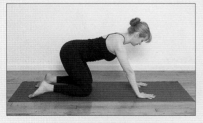

Four-point kneeling weight shift back

Finally, shift your weight in all directions. You can move circularly or diagonally. Notice how this changes the weight-bearing in your wrists. If you like, you can pause at any point where it feels good to experience additional stretch or load. Next, change the position of your hands. They can be closer together or further away from one another. You can also make your fingers point in a different direction. Start to shift your weight in all directions as you explore this new hand placement.

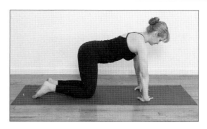

Four-point kneeling weight shift with fingers oriented towards one another

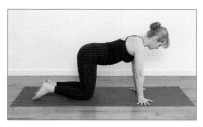

Four-point kneeling weight shift with fingers oriented away from one another

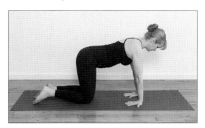

Four-point kneeling weight shift with fingers oriented towards knees

Four-point kneeling hip flexion peeling palms up from the floor with elbows straight

Come onto your hands and knees. Walk your hands forward, so they are slightly in front of your shoulders.

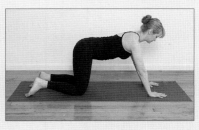

Four-point kneeling peeling palms up starting position

Maintaining elbow and finger extension, shift your hips towards your heels and peel your hands away from the floor into wrist extension.

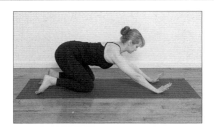

Four-point kneeling rock back with wrist extension

For additional challenge, you can practice this with your hands closer to your knees. Rock forward to return to the starting position. Perform five rounds.

Re-Check: Prayer palms "V" versus "T."

The next direction of movement to consider is hip flexion. Hip flexion occurs when the femur moves anteriorly or towards the chest, for example when sitting in a chair or moving into Forward Fold with a neutral spine. Many people will be limited in hip flexion, only performing it to get in and out of a chair, with the maximum movement being the distance from standing to sitting in a chair with knee flexion. Also, the movement form is typically passive and doesn't require strength or control, due to the support from the chair. Finally, many people sit with a posterior pelvic tilt, or their pelvis tucked under, which requires even less hip flexion.

Downward Facing Dog requires a significant amount of hip flexion with knee extension and a neutral pelvis, another reason why students may struggle with this pose. Associated movement compensations include:

- A posterior pelvic tilt
- An inability to straighten the knees
- Excessive spinal flexion

Below is an example sequence to address these movement compensations and build competency around hip flexion.

Hip flexion for Downward Facing Dog

Supine knee to chest

Lie on your back with your knees bent and your feet on the floor.

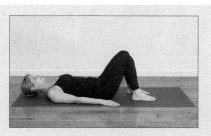

Supine knee to chest starting position

Without using your hands for assistance, bring your right knee towards your chest. Only move as far as you can go while maintaining a neutral spine and pelvis.

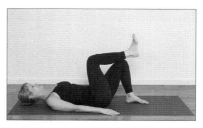

Supine knee to chest with right knee in hip flexion

Perform five rounds and repeat on the second side.

Supine marching in tabletop with resistance band around feet

Lie on your back with your knees bent and your feet flat on the floor. Bring your legs into a tabletop position. Place a light resistance loop band around the arches of your feet and dorsiflex your ankles.

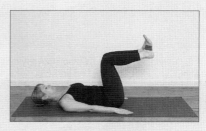

Supine marching with resistance band starting position

Hold your left leg still and maintain a neutral spine as you reach your right heel towards the floor.

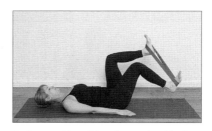

Supine marching with resistance band heel tap

Return to the starting position and repeat on the second side. Perform five rounds.

Supine straight leg to the sky

Lie on your back with your knees bent and your feet flat on the floor. Bring your right leg into a tabletop position with your right ankle in dorsiflexion.

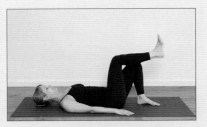

Supine single straight leg to the sky starting position

Maintain a neutral pelvis as you extend your right knee, so your heel reaches towards the sky. Bend your right knee to return to the starting position.

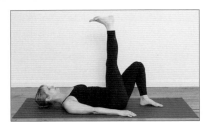

Supine single straight leg to the sky with knee extension

Perform five rounds and repeat on the second side.

To progress the exercise, practice this movement with both legs in tabletop position or both knees extended towards the ceiling.

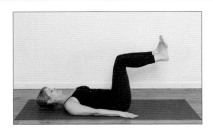

Supine both legs to sky starting position

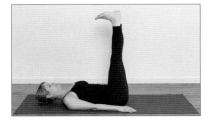

Supine both legs to sky with knee extension

The final direction of movement required for Downward Facing Dog is ankle dorsiflexion. Ankle dorsiflexion occurs when the foot is pulled back, so the toes move towards the shinbone. Many of our students will have limitations in dorsiflexion, because modern daily life requires very little of it. The most dorsiflexion the average person may need outside of the yoga studio is when they transition between sitting and standing. This is significantly less than the dorsiflexion required for Downward Facing Dog.

Students who lack the dorsiflexion needed for Downward Facing Dog commonly compensate for the lack of movement by distributing a significant amount of weight on to their arms. Once I have identified this, I will then select exercises to address ankle dorsiflexion.

Ankle dorsiflexion for Downward Facing Dog

Supine unilateral hamstring stretch

Lie on your back with your knees bent and your feet flat on the floor. Bring your right leg into tabletop. Place a yoga strap or resistance band around the ball of your right foot, holding the ends in your hands, and dorsiflex your ankle.

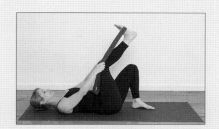

Supine unilateral hamstring stretch

Maintain ankle dorsiflexion and a neutral pelvis as you extend your right knee to reach your right heel towards the sky.

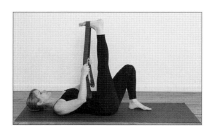

Supine unilateral hamstring stretch with knee extension

Bend your right knee to return to the starting position. Only extend your knee as far as you can while maintaining a neutral pelvis. Perform five rounds. Repeat this movement on the left side.

"The Thinker" with weight shifting

Come into a kneeling position. Take your right foot forward, so it connects to the floor. Keeping your chest connected to your right thigh, reach your arms forward. Notice how this will send your right knee past your right toes and will increase the load on your right foot.

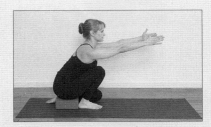

"The Thinker" with weight shifting starting position

Next, try lifting your buttocks off your left heel.

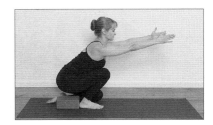

"The Thinker" with weight shifting lifting buttocks off heel

Experiment with shifting your weight in different directions over your right foot.

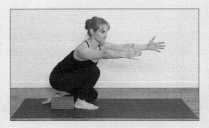

"The Thinker" with weight shifting right

Notice how it feels to practice this with your knee aligning over your second and third toe versus when it aligns with your little toe or big toe. Repeat on the second side.

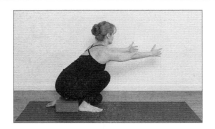

"The Thinker" with weight shifting left

"The Thinker" with ankle dorsiflexion and plantar flexion

Come into a kneeling position. Take your right foot forward, so it connects to the floor. Keeping your chest connected to your right thigh, reach your arms forward. As you lean your weight forward, push your right foot into the ground as if you are pressing the gas pedal in the car. Hold the contraction for 10–20 seconds and then release. Next, attempt to peel your toes and the top of your foot away from the ground without actually doing so. Note, this is an isometric contraction, so the position will not change. Hold the contraction for 10–20 seconds and then release. Perform three to five rounds and repeat on the second side.

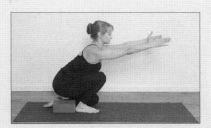

"The Thinker" with ankle dorsiflexion and plantar flexion

While the above example was specific to Downward Facing Dog, any pose can be deconstructed by identifying the directions of movement required at each joint, and then using these to pick preparatory exercises for your classes.

Teacher consideration

Choose a pose that is not Downward Facing Dog. What are the directions of movement required for that pose? Can you think of any compensatory movement patterns that you might see if your students have limitations in any of the directions of movement that you listed?

How to select preparatory exercises for more complicated poses

I used Downward Facing Dog as the example for this chapter because the pose is so linear and there are only four primary directions of movement. However, many poses are more complicated, and will require choosing preparatory exercises that relate to each aspect of the pose, based on the directions of movement required. From there, you can select exercises or create regressed versions of the pose, based on the principles discussed in Chapter 2.

For example, it would be difficult to find a preparatory exercise that directly matches the shape of Half Lord of the Fishes Pose (Ardha Matsyendrasana), because it involves spinal rotation with internal and external hip rotation, which are multiple directions of movement. For this pose, you could include one preparatory exercise emphasizing spinal rotation and another for internal and external hip rotation. From there, you could select exercises based on the principles of progression.

Chapter 8 provides more resources and ideas for preparatory exercises, including several sequences that build up to a single peak sequence or peak pose.

How to use preparatory exercises as a check/recheck for mini sequences within a class

When designing a class, I will often create or select multiple mini sequences emphasizing the directions of movement at the joints that are required for a final peak pose or peak sequence.

These mini sequences could include:

- A somatic sequence or sensory feedback method sequence

- A preparatory exercise sequence in supine

Chapter 7

- A preparatory exercise sequence in side lying

- A preparatory exercise sequence in prone

- A preparatory exercise sequence in four-point kneeling

- A preparatory exercise sequence in tall kneeling

- A preparatory exercise sequence in standing

- A preparatory exercise sequence in seated

(Please note that while I recommend sequencing classes in this order, you can switch the mini standing sequence and the mini seated sequence around.)

For each of these mini sequences, a single preparatory exercise might act as a check/recheck which I will choose based on the directions of movement that occur at each joint during the mini sequence. For example, if the somatic sequence that I intend to teach includes spinal extension and rotation, then I might choose preparatory exercises that emphasize spinal extension and rotation, so students can sense how the preparatory exercise now feels easier. When I teach the preparatory exercise as the check/recheck, I will also mention how this exercise teaches a movement skill required for the peak pose mini sequence that will take place at the end of class.

Preparatory exercises for Half Lord of the Fishes Pose

Spinal rotation: Supine roll and reach

Perform a check by assuming Half Lord of the Fishes Pose. Notice any sensation that you might experience across the shoulders and upper back.

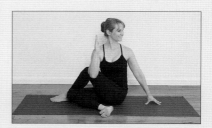

Half Lord of the Fishes pose

Lie on your back with your knees bent and your feet flat on the floor. Bring both arms out to shoulder height and let them rest on the ground with your palms facing the ceiling.

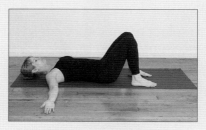

Supine roll and reach starting position

Bend your left elbow, so your left hand moves towards your chest.

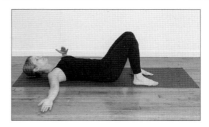

Supine roll and reach with left elbow bent

Continue to reach your left arm across your body, so your head and shoulders roll to the right. Try to keep your knees and pelvis still on the ground as you do this.

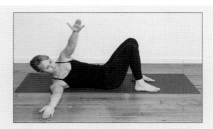

Supine roll and reach across the body

Reverse this movement to return to the starting position and repeat on the right side. Perform five rounds. Recheck Half Lord of the Fishes Pose and notice if you feel more ease in the pose.

Hip internal rotation: "The Betty Boop"

Lie on your back with your legs in tabletop position. Place a block between your knees with your legs parallel.

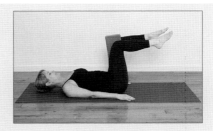

"The Betty Boop" starting position

Hug the block with your knees as you internally rotate your hips.

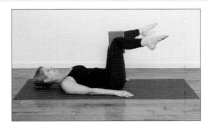

"The Betty Boop" with hip internal rotation

Externally rotate your hips to return to the starting position. Perform 10 to 12 repetitions.

Hip external rotation: Double supine clamshells

Lie on your back with your legs in tabletop position. Place a light to medium looped resistance band around your thighs.

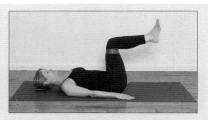

Double supine clamshells starting position

Press your heels together and externally rotate your thigh bones to make a frog position.

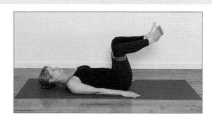

Double supine clamshells with hip abduction

Slowly return your legs to a tabletop position, so your thigh bones are parallel to one another. Maintain a neutral pelvis throughout the movement. Perform 10 to 12 repetitions.

To progress the exercise, practice it with a cork brick between your heel bones.

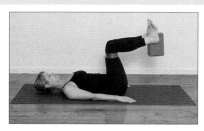

Double supine clamshells with block starting position

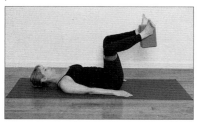

Double supine clamshells with block and hip abduction

To regress the exercise, practice it with your lower back imprinted into the floor.

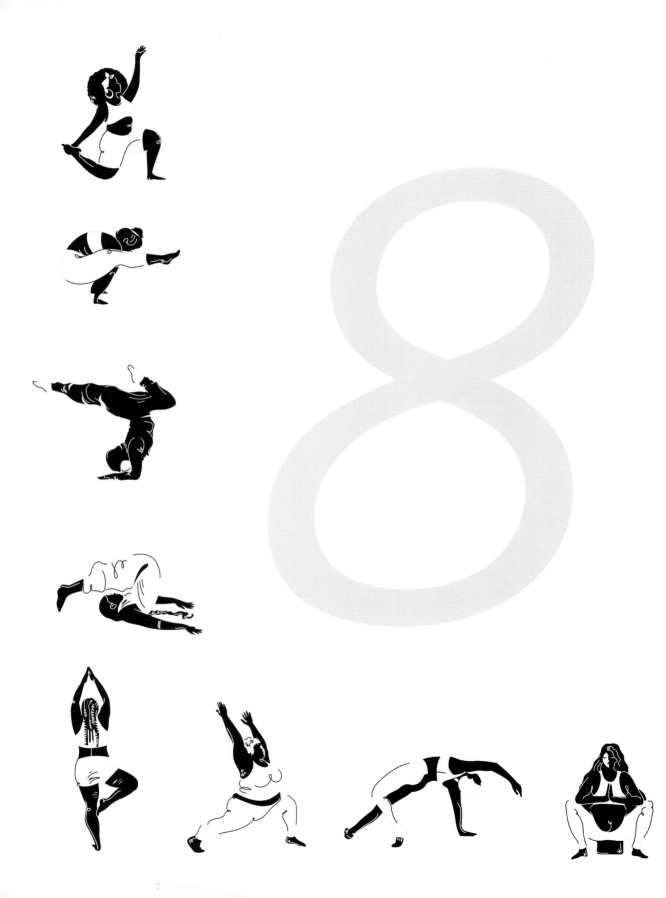

How to design a Yoga Deconstructed® class

Creating a Yoga Deconstructed class

When I create classes, each of them includes the following sequences in the order outlined below:

1. A variation of constructive rest

2. A sensory feedback method or somatic sequence

3. Preparatory exercises in supine, prone, or side lying

4. Preparatory exercises in kneeling or seated

5. Preparatory exercises in standing

6. A movement sequence that incorporates more traditional yoga poses

7. Savasana

You will notice that these sequences and concepts relate to the earlier chapters of this book.

There are many benefits to sequencing classes this way. Teaching in this order can help students connect to their deep stabilizing muscles and better prepare their bodies for traditional yoga poses. Additionally, it scales the exercises, so the most challenging movements happen near the end of class and students have an opportunity to opt out of a movement and pick a regression that was taught earlier. Finally, sequencing classes in this way provides an experience of mindfulness and flow, even if some of the movements aren't traditional yoga asanas.

How to use the template in this chapter

The template I've provided includes sequences to help you create your own classes using the methodology outlined in this book. While every class addresses the entire body, each class builds up to a peak pose that emphasizes the spine, lower body, or upper body, and includes a series of regressions and progressions to prepare the body for the final pose.

This template uses tracks. Each track includes sequences that correspond with both the class emphasis and a peak pose.

- Track 1: A variation of constructive rest

- Track 2: A sensory feedback method or somatic sequence

- Track 3: Preparatory exercises in supine, prone, or side lying

- Track 4: Preparatory exercises in seated or kneeling

- Track 5: Preparatory exercises in standing

- Track 6: A movement sequence to incorporate more traditional yoga poses

The sequences in Track 1 will apply to all classes. Tracks 2 through 6 each have three sections, which include sequences that have a specific class emphasis:

- Section 1: Spine

- Section 2: Lower body

- Section 3: Upper body

To create a class, decide if you would like to emphasize the spine, upper body, or lower body. Refer to the appropriate track and section. Select one sequence from each track. Teach each of these sequences in the order of their track numbers and you will have a complete class that begins with a variation of constructive rest and builds up to a peak pose. Each class will be approximately 60 to 75 minutes in length. While I didn't include instructions for Savasana, I recommend ending the class with it or another restorative pose.

Track 1 Constructive rest (interoception)

Ardha Savasana

1. Lie on your back with knees bent, feet flat on the floor, and hands placed on side ribs. Eyes can be closed to promote internal awareness, or you can pick a spot on the ceiling to focus on.

2. Mentally scan your body. Notice the weight of your head, shoulder blades, rib cage, pelvis, and feet on the floor.

3. Notice the circumferential expansion of your rib cage as your inhale. Allow yourself to surrender to gravity on the exhale. Perform up to five rounds of breathing.

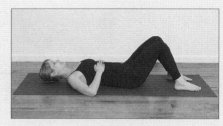

Ardha Savasana

Side-lying constructive rest

1. Lie on your side with knees bent. If needed, place a block under your head and a folded blanket between your knees for comfort. Place your top hand on the part of your rib cage that is facing the ceiling. Eyes can be closed to promote internal awareness, or you can pick a spot to focus on.

2. Mentally scan your body. Notice how your side body weights into the floor.

3. Notice the lateral expansion of your rib cage into your hand and the floor as you inhale. Allow yourself to surrender to gravity on the exhale. Perform up to five rounds of breathing.

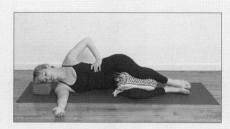

Side-lying constructive rest

Crocodile Pose

1. Lie facedown with hands resting on top of one another and your forehead on your hands. Place a folded blanket or block across your mid back for tactile feedback. Eyes can be closed to promote internal awareness.

2. Mentally scan your body. Notice how your belly expands into the floor and your back expands towards the ceiling as you inhale.

3. Allow yourself to soften into the floor as you exhale. Perform up to five rounds of breathing.

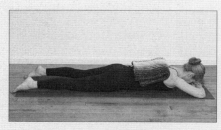

Crocodile Pose

Track 2 Sensory feedback methods and somatic sequences

Section 1 Spine emphasis

Ball-rolling sequence for the thoracic spine

1. Perform a check by assessing your spinal mobility with variations of Cat Cow. Gently move through flexion and extension. Notice where you feel the most movement versus where you feel the least movement. Do you feel the most or least movement in your lower back, middle back, or evenly throughout your spine?

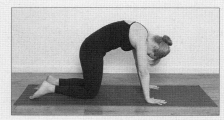

Cat Cow spinal flexion

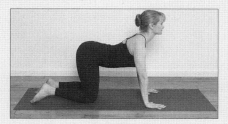

Cat Cow spinal extension

Repeat this process moving right to left through lateral flexion. Notice if you have more movement or access to breath in the right or left side.

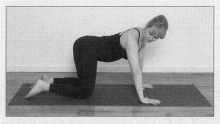

Cat Cow lateral flexion right

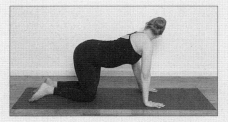

Cat Cow lateral flexion left

2. Lie on your back with one pinky ball on each side of the top of the medial border of the scapula and a yoga block underneath your sacrum. Arms should be down by your sides.

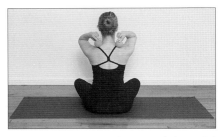

Pinky ball on each side of the top of the medial border of the scapula

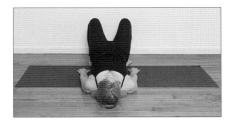

Ball rolling for the thoracic spine starting position

3. Reach your arms overhead into shoulder flexion. Notice how this increases the intensity of the feedback of the balls.

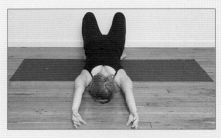

Ball rolling for the thoracic spine with shoulder flexion

Wave your arms so that your shoulder blades move through protraction, retraction, abduction, adduction, and circumduction. This will mimic a pin and stretch technique that is commonly used in massage therapy.

If you find a spot that feels good, you can pause in that place for a cycle of slower, deeper breaths.

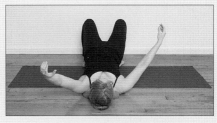

Example one of arm position when waving the arms

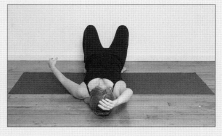

Example two of arm position when waving the arms

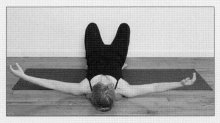

Example three of arm position when waving the arms

4. Remove the block and repeat step three with the balls halfway down the medial border of the scapula at about T5.

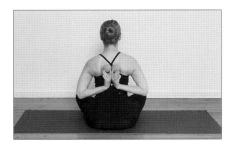

Ball placement at medial border of the scapula

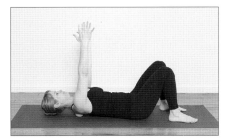

Scapular protraction

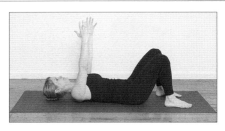

Scapular retraction

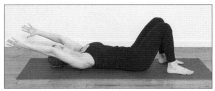

Shoulder flexion with balls at T5

5. Place the balls at the inferior border of the scapula at about T8.

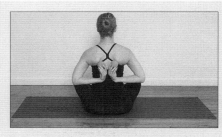

Balls at the inferior border of the scapula at T8

Hug yourself with your arms and gently roll side to side for five repetitions.

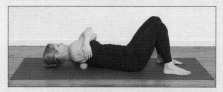

Hug yourself and roll side to side 1

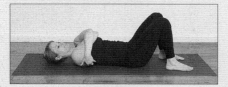

Hug yourself and roll side to side 2

6. Recheck by repeating the Cat Cow variations detailed in step one. Notice if you have more access to movement in the parts of your spine that felt stiff or if you feel more movement in your ribs when you breathe.

Ball-rolling sequence for the lumbar spine

1. Perform a check by assessing your spinal mobility with Jathara Parivartanasana (Revolved Abdomen Pose). Lie on your back with your knees tucked in towards your chest and your arms extended out to the sides at roughly shoulder height.

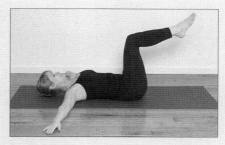

Revolved Abdomen Pose starting position

Float your legs to the left and notice your range of motion in rotation and any stretch that might occur in your lumbar spine.

Repeat on the right. Notice if you feel more stretch or have greater range of motion on one side.

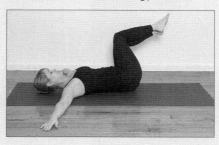

Revolved Abdomen Pose ending position

2. Lie on your back with knees bent and feet flat on the floor wider than hip width.

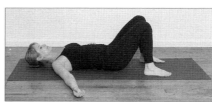

Lie supine

Place two balls in a vertical orientation on the right side of your lumbar spine near L5, S1 and T12, L1.

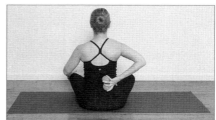

Balls to one side of lumbar spine near L5, S1 and T12, L1

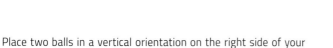

3. Laterally shift your pelvis right and left, and repeat on the left side of the lumbar spine.

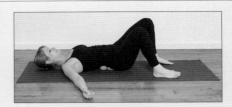

Laterally shift your pelvis right

Laterally shift your pelvis left

4. Place the balls in a horizontal configuration on the right and left side of your lumbar spine just above the superior aspect of the iliac crest.

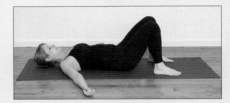

Ball placement above the superior aspect of the iliac crest

Interlace your fingers behind your right thigh and pull your thigh towards your chest to posteriorly tilt the pelvis and bring the lumbar spine into flexion.

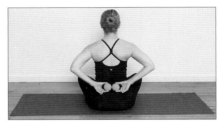

Pull your thigh towards your chest

Straighten your elbows to move your thigh away from your chest to anteriorly tilt the pelvis and bring the lumbar spine into extension.

Slowly alternate between these positions for five cycles and repeat on the left side.

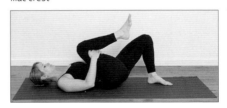

Move your thigh away from your chest

5. Recheck by repeating Jathara Parivartanasana (Revolved Abdominal Pose) as detailed in step one. Notice if you feel more ease in rotation and breath or less tension around the lumbar spine.

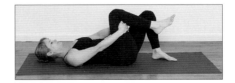

Somatic sequence: side-lying palm to palm

1. Perform a check by assessing your range of motion in thoracic rotation. Lie on your back with knees bent and feet flat on the floor wider than hip width. Place a block on your sternum and wrap your arms around yourself to secure it.

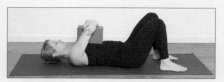

Thoracic rotation check starting position

Rotate your head and rib cage to the left, so your left shoulder blade leaves the ground. Try to keep your pelvis grounded and level.

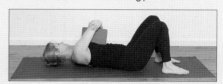

Rotate your head and ribcage left

Return to center and repeat on the right side.

Perform five cycles and notice if it was easier to rotate to one side versus the other.

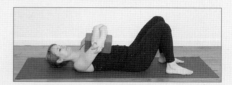

Rotate your head and ribcage right

2. Lie on your right side with your arms in front of you at shoulder height with palms facing each other and blanket under your head. Bend your knees to a 90-degree angle and place a block between your knees.

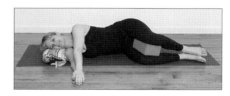

Side lying with arms at shoulder height

Slide your left hand forward, so it reaches beyond your right fingertips to touch the floor. Allow your chest and head to roll forward towards the floor.

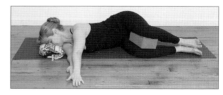

Slide your left hand forward

Keeping your left elbow straight, slide your left arm back, so your left hand slides along your right forearm. Allow your chest and head to roll back towards the ceiling. By keeping your elbow straight, you can isolate thoracic rotation.

Perform five rounds.

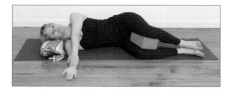

Slide your left arm back

3. Staying on your right side, angle both arms slightly downward towards your knees and repeat the movements outlined in step two for five rounds.

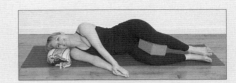

Side lying with arms angled down

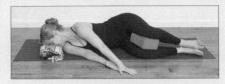

Slide left hand forward with arms angled down

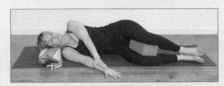

Slide left arm back with arms angled down

4. Next, angle both arms slightly upwards and repeat the same sequence outlined in step two for five rounds.

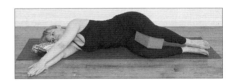

Side lying arms angled up

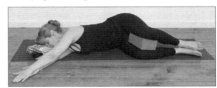

Slide left hand forward with arms angled up

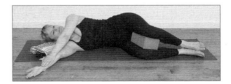

Slide left arm back with arms angled up

5. Repeat steps two through four on the left side.

6. Recheck by repeating the check outlined in step one. Notice if your range of motion has changed or if you feel more ease of movement.

Somatic sequence: prone salutes

1. Perform a check by assessing your range of motion in cervical and thoracic extension while in Crocodile Pose.

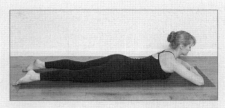

Crocodile Pose check

2. Lie facedown with your right hand resting on top of your left and your forehead resting on top of your hands.

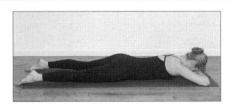

Lie prone

Keeping your head and hands still, slowly lift and lower your right elbow off the floor for five rounds. Notice how this affects the movement of your scapula.

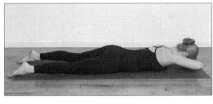

Place your left hand on top of your right and repeat this on the left side.

Lift and lower one elbow

3. Lie facedown with your left hand resting on top of your right and your forehead resting on top of your hands. Keeping your forehead connected to your left hand, slowly lift your left arm and head off the floor five times.

Place your right hand on top of your left and repeat this movement on the right side.

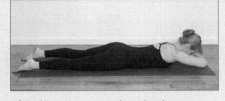

Lift and lower one arm and your head

Lie facedown with your right hand resting on top of your left and your forehead resting on top of your hands. Keeping your forehead connected to your right hand, slowly lift your right arm and head off the floor as you rotate your head and chest to the right.

Lower with control. Perform this movement five times. Place your left hand on top of your right and repeat this movement on the left side.

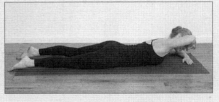

Lift and lower your upper body with rotation

4. Lie facedown with your left hand resting on top of your right and your forehead resting on top of your hands. Keeping your forehead connected to your hands, slowly lift both arms and your head off the floor. Keep the range of motion small enough that your bottom front ribs stay connected to the floor.

Lower with control. Perform this movement five times.

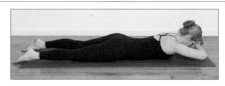

Lift and lower both arms

5. Recheck by repeating Crocodile Pose as outlined in step one. Notice if your range of motion has changed or if you feel more ease of movement.

Section 2 Lower-body emphasis

Ball-rolling sequence for the posterior aspect of the pelvis

1. Perform a check by assessing range of motion in hip external rotation using the figure four stretch. Lie on your back and cross your right ankle above your left knee. Interlace your fingers behind your left thigh and bring your legs towards your chest. Notice your range of motion and sensation around the posterior aspect of your right leg. Repeat on your left leg.

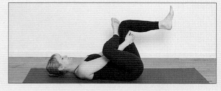

Figure four check

2. Lie on your back with your knees bent and your feet on the floor wider than hip width.

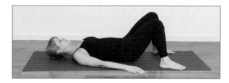

Lie supine

Place two balls in a vertical orientation at the lateral border of your left sacrum.

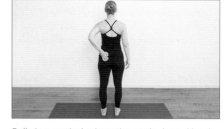

Balls in a vertical orientation at the lateral border of your left sacrum

Laterally shift your pelvis to the right and abduct your left leg, so the balls move towards the greater trochanter.

Reverse the movement to return to the starting position. Perform this movement for five rounds and repeat on the right side. To modify, perform this movement standing against a wall.

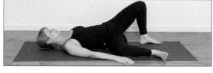

Laterally shift your pelvis to the right and abduct your left leg

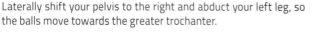

3. Lie on your right side and place two balls below the superior border of the right iliac crest with your right knee extended and your left knee bent with your foot flat on the floor behind your right.

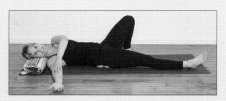

Side lying with balls below the superior border of the iliac crest

Pick up your left foot and place it in front of your right leg as your torso rotates towards the floor to move the balls anteriorly.

Pick up your left foot and place it behind your right leg as your torso rotates towards the ceiling to move the balls posteriorly. Perform for five rounds and repeat on the second side.

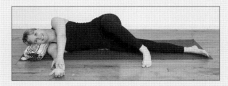

Pick up your left foot and place it in front of your right leg

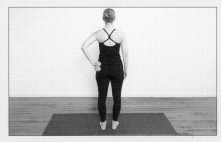

Ball placement when side lying with balls below the superior border of the iliac crest

4. Recheck by repeating the figure four stretch as outlined in step one. Notice if your range of motion in hip external rotation has improved.

Ball-rolling sequence for the anterior thigh

1. Perform a check by assessing range of motion in hip extension through Half Apanasana (Knee to Chest Pose). Lie on your back with your knees bent, feet flat on the floor, and a yoga block under your sacrum. Interlace your fingers behind your right thigh and bring your right knee towards your chest. Straighten your left knee and, if possible, ground your left heel into the floor. Notice the range of motion in your left hip and any sensation that you feel in the front of your left thigh. Repeat on the right and notice how it feels and if the sides are different from one another.

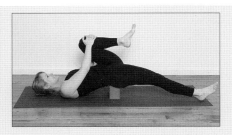

Hip extension check

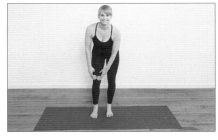

Ball placement with balls above patella

2. Lie prone with two balls in a horizontal configuration slightly above your right patella.

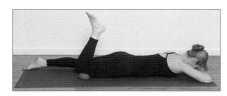

Prone with balls above right patella

Bend and straighten your right knee five times.

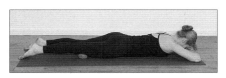

Bend and straighten your knee

3. Move balls halfway up the front of the right thigh in a vertical configuration.

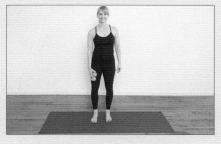

Vertical ball placement halfway up right thigh

Bend and straighten your knee five times.

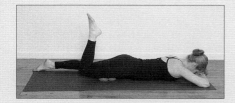

Bend and straighten your knee

Bend your right knee and move the thigh bone through internal and external rotation for five rounds.

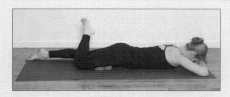

Internally rotate your thigh

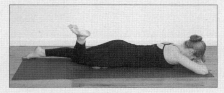

Externally rotate your thigh

4. Move the balls to the upper third of the right thigh in a horizontal configuration. Be mindful that the balls are below your hip crease.

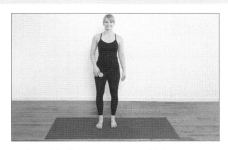

Horizontal ball placement upper thigh

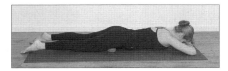

Balls at upper thigh with knee extended

Bend and straighten your right knee.

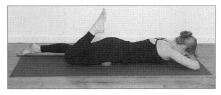

Balls at upper thigh with knee bent

5. Repeat steps two through four on the left thigh.

6. Recheck by repeating Half Apanasana (Knee to Chest Pose) as outlined in step one. Notice if your range of motion in hip extension has improved.

Somatic sequence: knee drops and slides

1. Perform a check by assessing range of motion in hip external rotation through figure four stretch. Lie on your back and cross your right ankle above your left knee. Interlace your fingers behind your left thigh and bring your legs towards your chest. Notice your range of motion and sensation around the posterior aspect of your right leg.

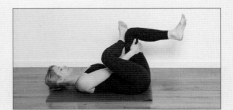

Figure four check

2. Lie on your back with knees bent and feet flat on the floor with feet about the width of your mat.

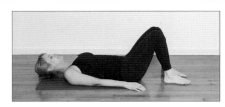

Lie supine

Allow your right knee to open to the right.

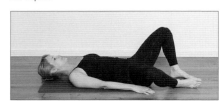

Allow your right knee to open to the right

Next, extend your right knee.

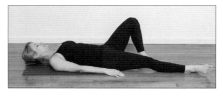

Right knee extended

Rotate your thigh to parallel.

Bend your right knee to return to the starting position. Next, allow your knee to fall in towards the midline, as you extend your right knee. Externally rotate your hip as you bend your right knee to return to the starting position. Perform five rounds and repeat on the left side.

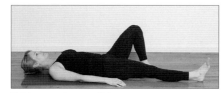

Thigh rotated to parallel

3. Recheck by repeating figure four stretch. Notice if your range of motion has changed or if you feel more ease of movement.

Somatic sequence: knee reach over toes

1. Perform a check by assessing range of motion in pelvic rotation. Lie on your back with knees bent and feet on the floor, sit bone-distance apart. Place an inflatable ball between your inner thighs. (If you do not have an inflatable ball, then you can use a rolled-up yoga mat or blanket instead.)

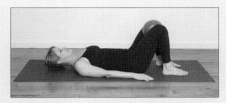

Supine with ball between thighs

Keeping both of your knees parallel and your feet grounded, reach your right knee over your right toes, so the left side of your pelvis becomes more weighted on the floor.

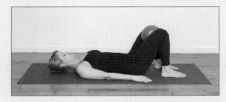

Reach your right knee over your right toes

Return to the starting position and repeat on the other side.

Perform five rounds and notice if you have more ease of movement or rotation on one side.

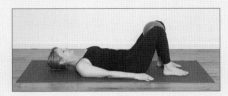

Reach left knee over left toes

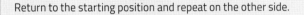

2. Lie on your back with your left knee bent and left foot flat on the floor and your right leg extended.

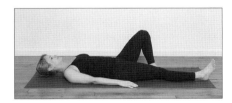

Lie supine with one knee extended

Push into your left foot and reach your left knee over your left toes, so your pelvis rotates to the right and the front of your left hip extends.

Return to starting position. Perform five rounds and repeat on the second side.

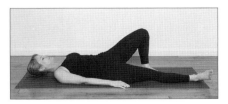

Rotate your pelvis right

3. Recheck by repeating the sequence outlined in step one. Notice if your range of motion has changed or if you feel more ease of movement.

Chapter 8

Ball-rolling sequence for trapezius and rotator cuff

1. Perform a check by assessing your range of motion at the gleno-humeral joint using controlled articulation in circumduction. Come into Virasana Pose, using props as needed for comfort. For example, you can sit on a yoga block or a blanket to elevate your pelvis.

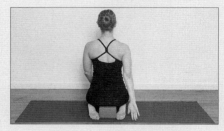

Virasana Pose

Reach your right arm towards the ceiling into shoulder flexion and external rotation. Pause and notice how much range of motion you have in this position.

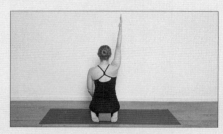

Shoulder flexion and external rotation

Next, internally rotate and extend your right shoulder to bring your arm behind you and close to your midline. Pause and notice how much range of motion you have in this position. Then, let your right arm rest by your side. Reverse this movement on the right side. Repeat the entire sequence on the left side.

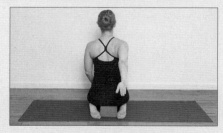

Shoulder internal rotation and extension with arm close to midline

2. Place the balls at the superior medial angle of the right and scapulas.

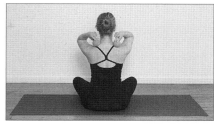

Ball placement superior medial angle of the right and left scapula

Lie on your back with knees bent and feet on the floor. Position a block horizontally underneath your sacrum on the lowest setting.

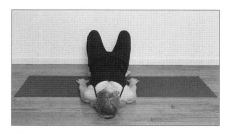

Lie supine with block under sacrum and balls at superior medial angle of scapula

3. Reach your arms overhead by your ears, so they rest on the floor.

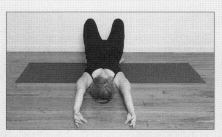

Shoulder flexion with balls at superior medial angle of scapula

To modify, bring them into a wider position. Pause and take a few breaths. Gently, roam your arms around in space and notice the sensation that the balls create when you move.

If you find an area that could use additional attention, then pause and breathe in that position.

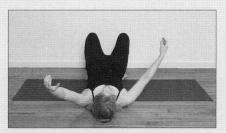

Move arms through space

4. Remove the block from under your pelvis. Then, take two balls and place them along the lateral border of your right scapula.

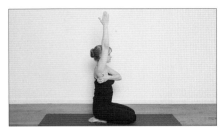

Ball placement lateral border of scapula

Reach your right arm overhead. Roll onto your right side.

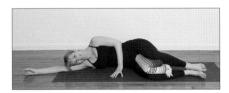

Side lying with balls at lateral border of scapula

Gently, roll your torso forward and back to massage the balls along this area five times.

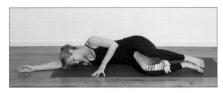

Roll torso forward

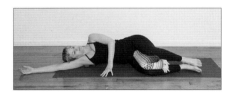

Roll torso backward

5. Lower your right arm to shoulder height, so it's in front of you. Place a block or blanket under your head for comfort. Bend your right elbow to 90 degrees, so your fingertips point up towards the ceiling.

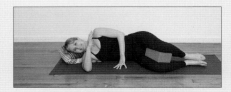

Side lying with elbow bent at 90 degrees

Keeping your elbow bent, lower the palm of your hand towards the floor, so your glenohumeral joint moves into internal rotation.

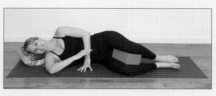

Glenohumeral internal rotation

Reverse the movement to bring your glenohumeral joint into external rotation. Repeat for five rounds.

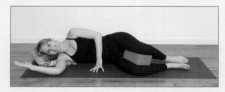

Glenohumeral external rotation

6. Repeat steps four through five on the left side.

7. Recheck by repeating Virasana Pose as outlined in step one. Notice if your range of motion has changed or if you feel more ease of movement.

Ball-rolling sequence for the upper chest

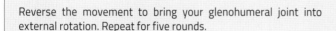

1. Perform a check by assessing your range of motion at the glenohumeral joint while in Crocodile Pose. Lie facedown with your hands resting on top of one another and your forehead on your hands. Abduct your right arm with your thumb facing the ceiling.

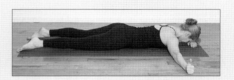

Lie prone

Hover your arm off the floor. Pause and notice how much range of motion you have in this position.

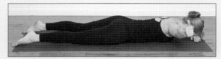

Hover arm off the floor

Next, reach your arm overhead into shoulder flexion.

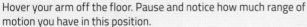

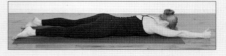

Arm reaching overhead

Hover your arm off of the floor. Pause and notice how much range of motion you have in this position.

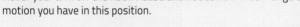

Sweep your arm between these two positions for five rounds and notice how it feels. Repeat on your left side.

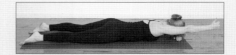

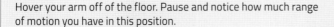

Arm hovered off the floor with shoulder flexion

2. Stack two yoga blocks. Kneel and position one ball below your right clavicle, adjacent to your sternum, so it is sandwiched between your chest and the yoga block. Place your hands on the ground for support and allow your head to hang.

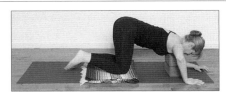

Ball between clavicle and stacked blocks

Shift your torso side to side, so the ball moves along your chest from sternum to shoulder.

Repeat for five rounds.

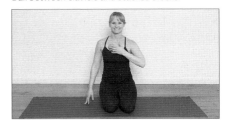

Ball position near sternum

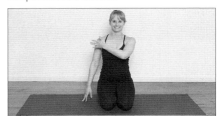

Ball position near shoulder

3. Move the ball, so it is below your right clavicle close to your shoulder and sandwiched between your chest and the yoga block.

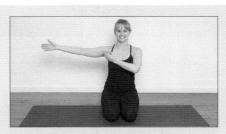

Ball position between chest and block

Abduct your right arm with your thumb facing the ceiling.

Next, reach your arm overhead into shoulder flexion. Sweep your arm between these two positions for five rounds to create a pin and stretch effect.

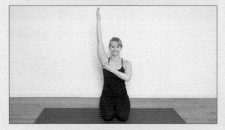

Ball position between chest and block with shoulder flexion

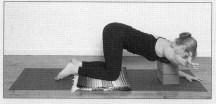

Ball between clavicle and stacked blocks with shoulder abduction

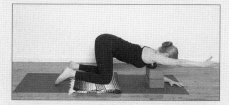

Ball between clavicle and stacked blocks with shoulder flexion

4. Repeat steps two and three on your left side.

5. Recheck by repeating Crocodile Pose as outlined in step one. Notice if your range of motion has changed or if you feel more ease of movement.

Somatic sequence: "X" rolls upper extremity

1. Perform a check by assessing your range of motion in thoracic rotation. Lie on your right side with your right arm at shoulder height, your left hand on your sternum, and blanket under your head. Bend your knees to a 90-degree angle and place a block between your knees.

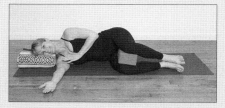

Side lying with block between knees and thumb at sternum

Keeping your left hand on your sternum, rotate your chest and head towards the ceiling.

Return to the starting position. Perform for five rounds and repeat on second side. Notice if you have more ease of movement or rotation on one side.

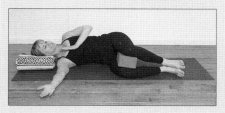

Side lying rotate backwards

2. Lie on your back with your arms resting on the floor overhead in a "V" with your legs straight and mat-width apart, so you are making an "X" shape with your body.

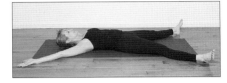

Lie supine with arms in a "V"

3. Slide your right arm along the floor towards your head. If possible, keep your elbow straight and your arm on the floor during this action.

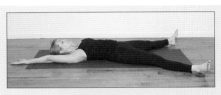

Slide your right arm along the floor towards your head

Next, turn your head to the left as you continue tracing the floor with your right fingers until your palms touch. Reverse the movement to return to the starting position. Perform five rounds and repeat on the second side.

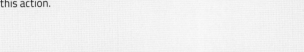

Turn your head as you trace the floor with your hand

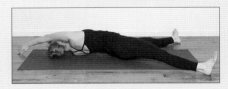

Continue to trace the floor in a circle

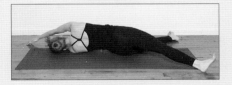

Reach your left hand towards your right

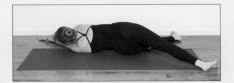

Bring your palms to touch

4. Recheck by repeating the sequence outlined in step one. Notice if your range of motion has changed or if you feel more ease of movement.

Somatic sequence: shoulder rotations

1. Perform a check by assessing your range of motion in gleno-humeral internal and external rotation. Lie on your back with knees bent, feet flat on the floor, and arms out to the sides at shoulder height. Make fists with your hands and place the pinkie side down on the floor. Internally rotate your shoulders, so your thumbs move towards the floor.

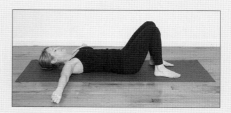

Internally rotate your shoulders

Reverse directions and externally rotate your shoulders. Perform five rounds and notice your range motion and ease of movement.

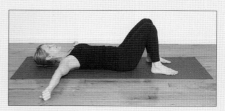

Externally rotate your shoulders

2. Lie on your back with knees bent, feet flat on the floor, and arms out to the sides at shoulder height. Make fists with your hands and place the pinkie side down on the floor. Tilt your head back, so your chin reaches gently towards the ceiling and your mid ribs get heavier on the floor. Allow your shoulders to internally rotate as you do this.

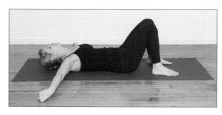

Tilt your head back

Return to the starting position and perform for five rounds. Next, nod your head forward, keeping the back of your head resting on the ground. As you do this, feel your mid ribs get lighter on the floor. Allow your shoulders to externally rotate as you do this. Return to the starting position and perform for five rounds.

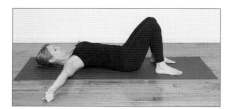

Nod your head forward

3. Recheck by repeating the sequence outlined in step one. Notice if your range of motion has changed or if you feel more ease of movement.

Track 3 Preparatory exercises in supine, prone, or side lying

Section 1 Spine emphasis

Spine emphasis sequence A

Bridge lifts with spinal articulation

1. Lie on your back with knees bent, feet flat on the floor, and a block between your inner thighs at the second setting.

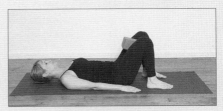

Lie supine with a block between your knees

2. Posteriorly tilt your pelvis and peel up through your spine to lift your hips towards the ceiling. As you do this, reach your arms overhead into shoulder flexion. See if you can lift your hips and arms at the same time.

3. Reverse directions and articulate through your spine to return to the starting position. See if you can connect your hands and hips to the floor at the same time. Perform five to eight repetitions.

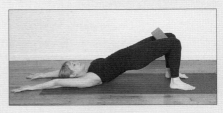

Bridge with shoulder flexion

Jathara Parivartanasana (Revolved Abdomen Pose)

1. Lie on your back with your ankles and knees touching in tabletop and your arms out to the sides in a "T" position.

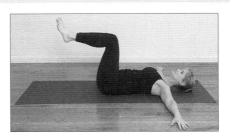

Tabletop legs

2. Take your legs to the right, while keeping your shoulder blades connected to the floor and your legs pressed together.

3. Return to starting position and repeat on the other side. Perform four to six sets.

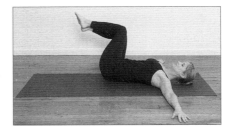

Tabletop legs to one side

Side bend slides

1. Set up for this exercise by unfolding a blanket. Fold the blanket in half lengthwise, so it looks like your yoga mat.

2. Lie on the blanket with your knees bent and your feet flat on the floor. Make sure that your head and your feet are on the blanket and not on the floor.

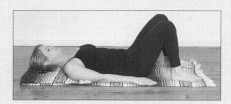

Lie supine on a blanket

3. Keeping your feet connected to the blanket, laterally flex your spine to the right, so your right shoulder moves towards your right hip and your spine makes a "C" shape. Be mindful that both of your shoulder blades and sides of your pelvis stay equally weighted on the blanket.

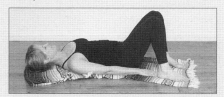

Laterally flex your spine right

4. Reverse directions to return to the starting position and repeat by side bending to the left. Perform four to six sets.

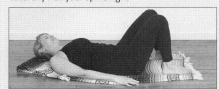

Laterally flex your spine left

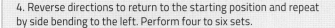

Spine emphasis sequence B

Roly poly

1. Lie on your right side with your arms in front of you at shoulder height with palms connected and hips and knees flexed at a 90-degree angle.

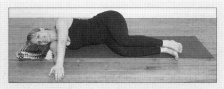

Side lying with arms at shoulder height

2. Lift your left arm and left leg up towards the ceiling. Abduct as far as you can without lifting the right arm and leg.

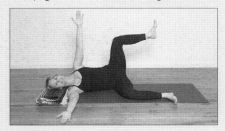

Arm and leg abduction

3. Lift the right arm and leg as you roll onto your left side, so you land in the same position you started in, except now the left side of your body is connected to the floor.

4. Perform four to six repetitions, alternating sides.

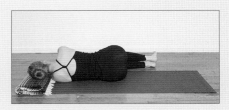

Roll to second side

Supine robot arms

1. Lie on your back with knees bent and feet flat on the floor. Bend your elbows to 90 degrees and make fists with your hands.

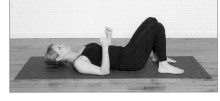

Lie supine with hands in fists

2. Press your elbows and head into the floor as you extend through your mid back. Release to the floor with control and allow your arms to come down by your sides.

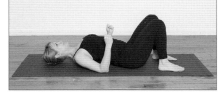

Mid back extension

3. Float your arms an inch off the floor and slowly lift your head to curl forward into flexion. Pause when your ribs are heavy and your shoulder blades are off the ground. Lower to the ground with control.

4. Alternate between the movements outlined in steps two and three for four to six rounds.

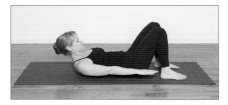

Spinal flexion with head lift

Rolling like a ball

1. Start in a seated position. Place your hands on the middle of your shins and round your spine into spinal flexion. Roll back just far enough that you can balance with your feet off the floor.

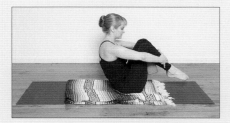

Seated spinal flexion with feet off the floor

2. Keeping your hands connected to your lower legs, rock back while maintaining spinal flexion.

3. When your shoulder blades touch the floor, rock forward to the starting position while maintaining spinal flexion with your feet off the floor. Perform up to eight repetitions.

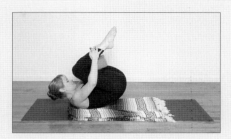

Roll back in spinal flexion

Rolling like a ball with a block

1. Start in a seated position with one block between the back of your thighs and your calves. Place your hands on the middle of your shins and round your spine into spinal flexion. Roll back just far enough that you can balance with your feet off the floor.

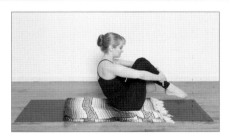

Seated spinal flexion with block and feet off the floor

2. Without dropping the block, rock back while maintaining spinal flexion.

3. When your shoulder blades touch the floor, rock forward to the starting position while maintaining spinal flexion. Perform up to eight repetitions.

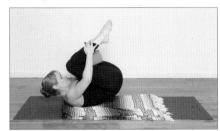

Roll back in spinal flexion with block

Section 2 Lower-body emphasis

Lower-body emphasis sequence A

Supine Half Moon with a strap

1. Lie on your back with your right leg straight on the floor and your left leg reaching towards the ceiling. Place a strap around your left foot and hold on to each end with your hands.

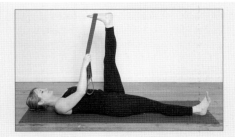

Lie supine with foot in strap

2. Keeping both sides of your pelvis equally weighted on the floor, abduct your left leg out to the side away from your midline.

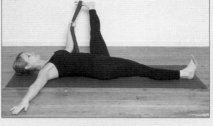

Foot in strap with leg abduction

3. Adduct your left leg towards the midline to return to the starting position. Try to keep your pelvis still and level as you perform this movement.

4. Perform five repetitions and repeat on the second side.

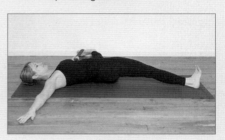

Be mindful not to shift onto one side of your pelvis as seen here

Supine Half Moon hovers

1. Lie on your back with your left leg straight on the floor, your arms out by your sides in a "T" position, and your right leg abducted to the side with your right calf resting on two blocks.

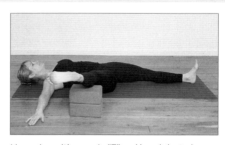

Lie supine with arms in "T" and leg abducted

2. Press your arms and left leg into the ground to hover your right leg off the blocks. Hold this position for five breaths, trying to keep both sides of the back of your pelvis equally weighted on the floor. Lower with control to return to the starting position.

3. Perform three to five repetitions and repeat on the second side.

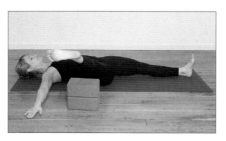

Leg hover off blocks with arms in "T"

Supine Half Moon to Warrior III

1. Lie on your back with your left leg straight on the floor, your arms reaching over your head, and your right leg abducted to the side with your right calf resting on two blocks.

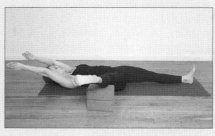

Lie supine with shoulder flexion and leg abducted

2. Press your left leg into the ground to lift your right leg off the block and up towards the ceiling, while keeping both sides of the back of your pelvis equally weighted on the floor. Lower with control to return to the starting position.

3. Perform three to five repetitions and repeat on the second side.

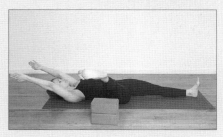

Leg hovers off blocks with shoulder flexion

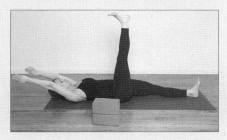

Leg to ceiling with shoulder flexion

Supine Half Moon to Warrior III with a strap

1. Lie on your back with your left leg straight on the floor and your right leg abducted to the side with your right calf resting on two blocks. Reach your arms up towards the ceiling and hold on to a strap with hands shoulder-width apart.

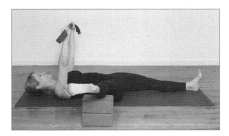

Lie supine with hands holding strap and leg abducted

2. Tug on the strap and externally rotate and depress your shoulders. Maintaining tension on the strap, press your left leg into the ground to lift your right leg off the block and up towards the ceiling, while keeping both sides of the back of your pelvis equally weighted on the floor. Lower with control to return to the starting position.

3. Perform three to five repetitions and repeat on the second side.

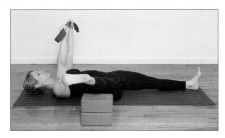

Leg hovers off block while hands hold strap

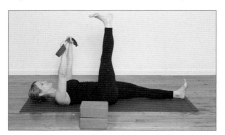

Leg to ceiling while hands hold strap

Lower-body emphasis sequence B

Active hamstring stretch

1. Lie on your back with your knees bent and feet flat on the floor. Bring your right knee to your chest and interlace your hands on the back of your right thigh. Check that you have a neutral pelvis.

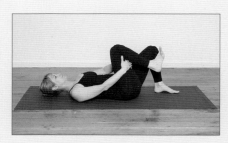

Hug knee to chest

2. Slowly bend and straighten your right knee, keeping your right thigh bone close to you and your pelvis level and still. As you straighten your knee, dorsiflex your right ankle.

3. Perform up to six repetitions and repeat on the second side.

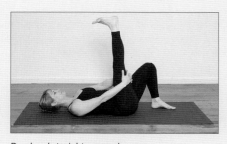

Bend and straighten your knee

Cook hip lift

1. Lie on your back with your knees bent and feet flat on the floor. Bring your right knee to your chest and interlace your hands on the front of your right shin.

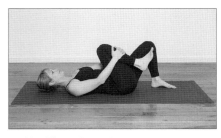

Cook hip lift starting position

2. Keeping your right knee close to your chest, press into your left foot to lift your hips off the ground. Try to keep your pelvis level as you do this.

3. Lower your hips with control. Perform eight repetitions and repeat on the second side.

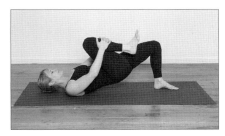

Cook hip lift ending position

Single leg bridge

1. Lie on your back with your knees bent and feet flat on the floor. Extend your right leg up to the ceiling and check that your pelvis is level and neutral. If you are unable to flex your hip to 90 degrees with your knee straight, bend your right knee to a 90-degree angle to modify.

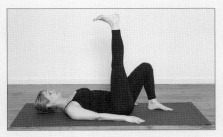

Single leg bridge starting position

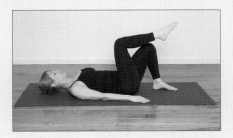

Bridge modification starting position

2. Press into your arms and your left foot to lift your pelvis off the floor. Try to keep your pelvis level and neutral as you do this.

3. Lower with control. Perform eight repetitions and repeat on the second side.

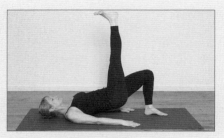

Single leg bridge ending position

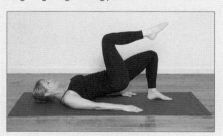

Bridge modification ending position

Section 3 Upper-body emphasis

Upper-body emphasis sequence A

Side-lying book openers

1. Lie on your right side with your right arm at shoulder height, your left hand behind your head, and a blanket under your head. Bend your knees to a 90-degree angle and place a block between your knees.

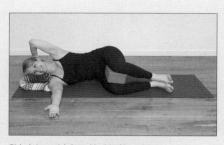

Side lying with hand behind head

2. Rotate your chest and head towards the ceiling. As you do this, try to keep your knees stacked and your pelvis still.

3. Return to the starting position. Perform for five rounds and repeat on the second side.

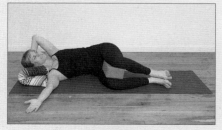

Rotate chest towards ceiling

Prone "T", "V", "I" lifts

1. Lie facedown with your forehead resting on a blanket for comfort. Reach your arms out to the sides in a "T" position and make fists with your thumbs facing the ceiling.

Hover your arms off the floor and hold for five breaths. Lower with control. Repeat one more time.

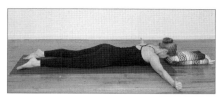

Prone with arms in "T"

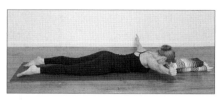

Hover arm off the floor in "T"

2. Reach your arms overhead in a "V" position and make fists with your thumbs facing the ceiling. Hover your arms off the floor and hold for five breaths. Lower with control. Repeat one more time.

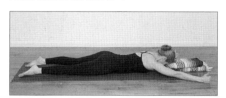

Prone with arms in "V"

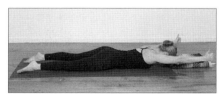

Hover arm off the floor in "V"

3. Narrow your arms overhead in an "I" position and make fists with your thumbs facing the ceiling. Hover your arms off the floor and hold for five breaths. Lower with control. Repeat one more time.

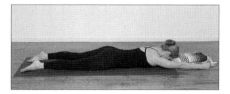

Prone with arms in "I"

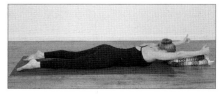

Hover arm off the floor in "I"

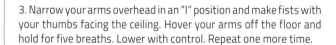

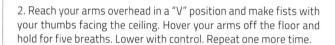

Prone Michael Phelps arms

1. Lie facedown with your forehead resting on a blanket for comfort. Place both hands behind your head with one hand resting on top of the other.

2. Hover both of your hands off your head.

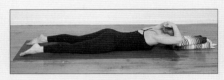

Prone with arms and head hovering

3. Sweep your arms out to a "T" and down by your sides, bending your elbows so your hands hover off your lower back. Try not to touch your torso with your hands as you do this.

4. Reverse directions to return to the starting position.

5. Perform three to five repetitions and repeat for one more set. For additional challenge, hover your head off the floor for the second set.

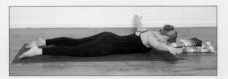

Sweep arms down by sides

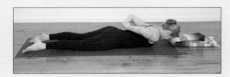

Bring arms behind back

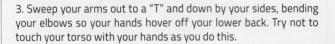
Upper-body emphasis sequence B

Arm circles

1. Lie lengthwise on a foam roller. If you do not have a foam roller, you can lie on a rolled-up yoga mat with your head resting on a folded blanket stacked on a block. If your pelvis is hanging off the rolled-up mat, place a block under your pelvis.

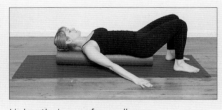

Lie lengthwise on a foam roller

2. Reach your arms up towards the ceiling.

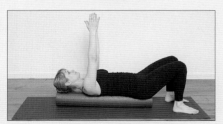

Reach your arms up towards the ceiling

3. Reach your arms overhead into shoulder flexion. Try to keep the back of your ribs heavy and your pelvis neutral on the rolled-up mat as you do this.

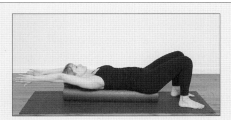

Reach your arms overhead into shoulder flexion

4. Open your arms out to the sides like a snow angel and reach your arms down by your hips.

5. Perform three to five arm circles and then reverse directions.

6. Repeat steps one through five holding cork blocks or hand weights to add load.

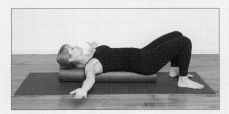

Arms opened out to sides

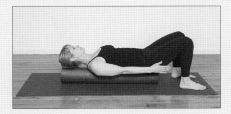

Reach your arms down by hips

Supine "T", "V", "I" lifts

1. Lie lengthwise on a rolled-up yoga mat with your head resting on a folded blanket stacked on a block. If your pelvis is hanging off the rolled-up mat, place a block under your pelvis.

2. Hold on to small hand weights or cork blocks and open your arms out to the sides in a "T" position with your palms facing the ceiling.

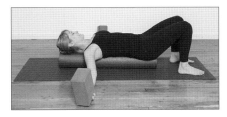

Arms in "T" with blocks

3. Keeping your elbows straight, hover your arms up to shoulder height. Hold for five breaths and lower with control. Keep the humeral head centrated in the glenoid fossa. Perform up to two sets.

To modify, perform without hand weights or cork blocks.

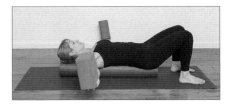

Arms hover in "T" with blocks

4. Reach your arms overhead in a "V" position and hold on to the hand weights or cork bricks with your pinkies facing the ceiling. Keeping the humeral head centrated in the glenoid fossa, hover your arms up to shoulder height and hold for five breaths. Lower with control. Repeat one more time.

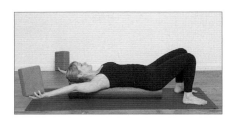

Arms in "V" with blocks

5. Narrow your arms overhead in an "I" position and hold on to the hand weights or cork bricks with your pinkies facing the ceiling. Keeping the humeral head centrated in the glenoid fossa, hover your arms up to shoulder height and hold for five breaths Lower with control. Repeat one more time.

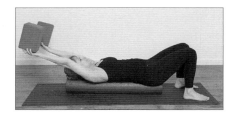

Arms in "I" with blocks

Side-lying arm circles

1. Lie on your right side with your arms in front of you at shoulder height and a blanket under your head. Flex your hips and knees to a 90-degree angle and place a block between your knees.

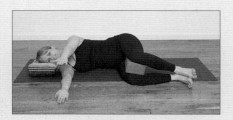

Side lying with arms at shoulder height

2. Flex and externally rotate your left shoulder, so your arm is by your ear. Pause and notice how much range of motion you have in this position.

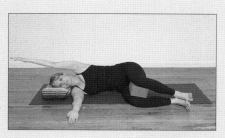

Flex and externally rotate your left shoulder

3. Internally rotate and extend your left shoulder to bring your arm behind you and close to your midline. Pause and notice how much range of motion you have in this position.

4. Rest your left arm on top of your hip. Reverse this movement on the left side.

5. Repeat the entire sequence on the right side.

6. Perform three to five arm circles and then reverse directions.

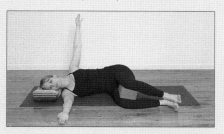

Internally rotate and extend your left shoulder (A)

7. Repeat steps one through six holding cork blocks or hand weights to add load.

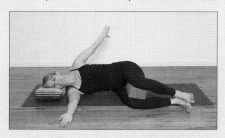

Internally rotate and extend your left shoulder (B)

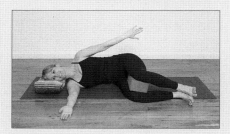

Internally rotate and extend your left shoulder (C)

Track 4 Preparatory exercises in kneeling or seated

Section 1 Spine emphasis

Spine emphasis sequence A

Serratus push-ups on forearms

1. Come into four-point kneeling with your knees under your hips and your elbows under your shoulders. Place your forearms parallel to each other on two blocks on the second setting.

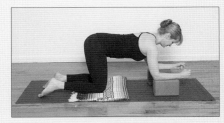

Four-point kneeling

2. Allow your sternum to lower towards the ground, so your shoulder blades move into retraction. Try to keep your spine neutral through the movement.

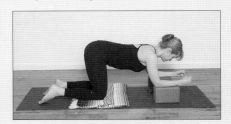

Four-point kneeling scapular retraction

3. Press into your forearms to lift your rib cage up towards the ceiling. This will create shoulder blade protraction. Try to keep your spine neutral through the movement.

4. Perform six to eight repetitions.

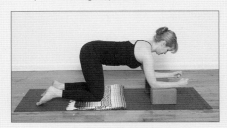

Four-point kneeling scapular protraction

Elevation and depression on forearms

1. Come into four-point kneeling with your knees under your hips and your elbows under your shoulders. Place your forearms parallel to each other on two blocks on the second setting.

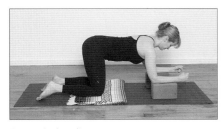

Four-point kneeling

2. Find a neutral spine and elevate your shoulder blades up to your ears.

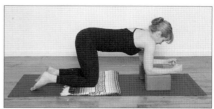

Four-point kneeling scapular elevation

3. Maintain a neutral spine as you depress your shoulder blades away from your ears.

4. Perform six to eight repetitions.

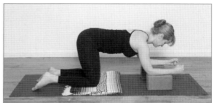

Four-point kneeling scapular depression

Scapula circles

1. Come into four-point kneeling with your knees under your hips and your elbows under your shoulders. Place your forearms parallel to each other on two blocks on the second setting.

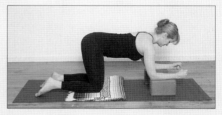

Four-point kneeling

2. Find a neutral spine and elevate your shoulder blades up to your ears.

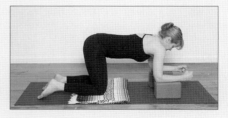

Four-point kneeling scapular elevation

3. Allow your sternum to lower towards the ground, so your shoulder blades move into retraction. Try to keep your spine neutral through the movement.

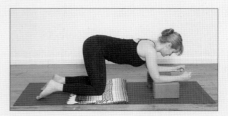

Four-point kneeling scapular retraction

4. Maintain scapular retraction as you depress your shoulder blades away from your ears.

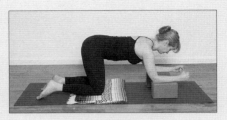

Four-point kneeling scapular depression

5. Press into your forearms to protract your shoulder and lift your rib cage up towards the ceiling.

6. Perform three to five repetitions. Then reverse directions.

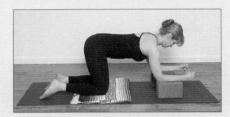

Four-point kneeling scapular protraction

Articulated Cat Cow

1. Come into four-point kneeling with your knees under your hips and your elbows under your shoulders. Place your forearms parallel to each other on two blocks on the second setting.

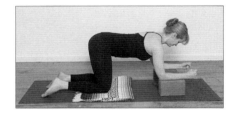

Four-point kneeling

2. Flex your spine. Make sure that you are in cervical flexion, lumbar flexion, and a posterior pelvic tilt.

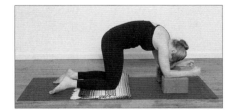

Four-point kneeling spinal flexion

3. Maintain cervical and thoracic flexion as you begin to anteriorly tilt your pelvis.

4. Allow the lumbar spine to move into extension while maintaining flexion in the segments above.

5. Slowly begin to extend your thoracic spine while maintaining cervical flexion.

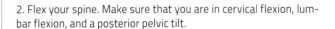

Four-point kneeling anterior pelvic tilt

6. Allow the cervical spine to move into extension, so you are in Cow Pose.

7. Reverse the movement with spinal articulation into flexion, beginning with the pelvis and ending with the cervical spine.

8. Perform three to five repetitions.

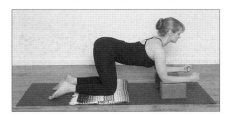

Four-point kneeling spinal extension

Look at your tail

1. Come into four-point kneeling with your knees under your hips and your elbows under your shoulders. Place your forearms parallel to each other on two blocks on the second setting.

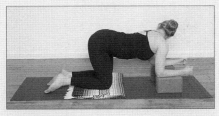

Four-point kneeling

2. Turn your head to the right and try to look at your outer right hip as you laterally flex your spine to the right.

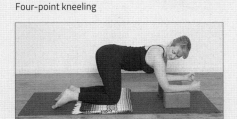

Lateral flexion right

3. Move through center to turn your head to the left and try to look at your outer left hip as you laterally flex your spine to the left.

4. Try to keep your pelvis stacked over your knees as you laterally flex right and left. Perform three to five repetitions.

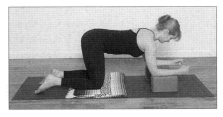

Lateral flexion left

Scrape the peanut butter

1. Come into four-point kneeling with your knees under your hips and your elbows under your shoulders. Place your forearms parallel to each other on two blocks on the second setting.

Four-point kneeling

2. Flex your spine to move into Cat Pose.

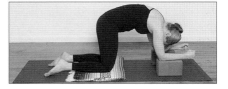

Four-point kneeling spinal flexion

3. Laterally flex your spine to the right.

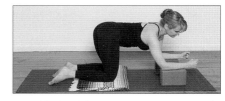

Lateral flexion right

4. Move through center to extend your spine in Cow Pose.

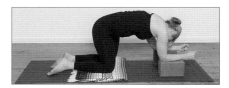

Transition through center

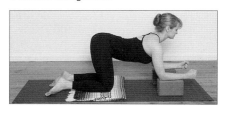

Four-point kneeling spinal extension

5. Laterally flex your spine to the left and return to Cat Pose.

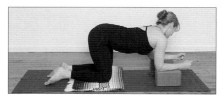

Lateral flexion left

6. Perform three to five repetitions and reverse directions.

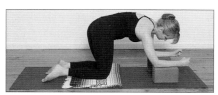

Four-point kneeling spinal flexion

Spine emphasis sequence B

Sliding thread the needle

1. Fold your mat in half to create padding for your knees. Come into four-point kneeling with your knees at the front edge of your mat and your left hand on a folded blanket in front of you.

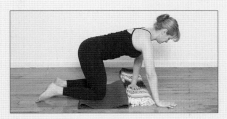

Four-point kneeling hand on blanket

2. Internally rotate your left arm and slide your left arm to the right as you bend your right elbow. Allow your chest to rotate to the right.

3. Straighten your right elbow to return to the starting position. Place your right hand on the blanket and repeat on the second side. Perform five sets, alternating sides.

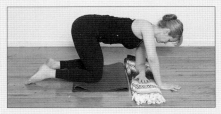

Internally rotate your left arm and slide your left arm to the right

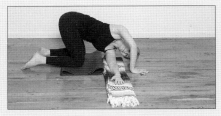

Allow your chest to rotate to the right

Gyroscopic swirls

1. Fold your mat in half to create padding for your knees and unfold a blanket. Gather the blanket together with your hands.

2. Come into four-point kneeling with your knees on the front edge of your mat and your hands on the edges of the blanket.

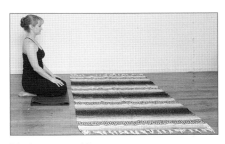

Blanket start position

3. Internally rotate your arms. Slide your right arm forward and to the left as your slide your left arm back and to the right, so your chest rotates to the right and your spine moves into flexion.

4. Return to center and repeat on the second side. Perform five sets, alternating sides each time.

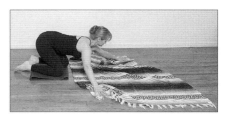

Gather the blanket with your hands

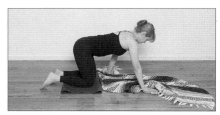

Four-point kneeling with hands on blanket

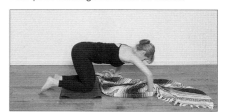

Internally rotate your arms

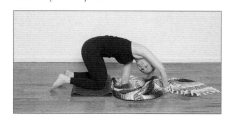

Slide your right arm forward and to the left as your slide your left arm back

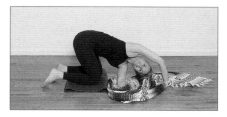

Rotate your chest and move into flexion

Tetris click the blocks

1. Come into a tall kneeling position and hold on to one block in each hand with your arms down by your sides. For additional challenge, use cork blocks.

2. Reach your arms out to the side and overhead and touch the ends of the blocks to one another.

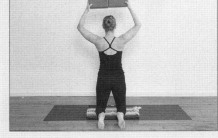

Touch the blocks overhead

3. Lower your arms and try to touch the ends of the blocks behind you. As you do this, try to lift your arms as high as you can.

4. Perform five sets. Try to keep your torso still and your pelvis and spine neutral as you move your arms.

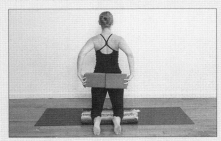

Touch the blocks behind you

Section 2 Lower-body emphasis

Lower-body emphasis sequence A

Take your triangle on a walk

1. Come into a seated straddle position.

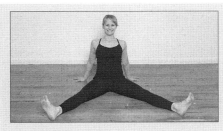

Sit in a straddle position

2. Shift your weight to the left and allow the left leg to move into external rotation as the right leg moves into internal rotation. Try to bring your left pinky toe and your right big toe to the ground as you do this. The right side of your pelvis will lift off the ground.

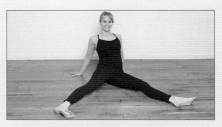

Shift your weight left and rotate your legs

3. Shift your weight to the center and repeat on the second side. For additional challenge, perform the movement with your hands off the ground.

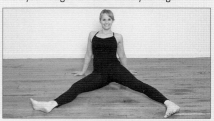

Shift your weight right and rotate your legs

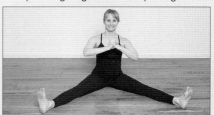

Take your triangle on a walk progression (A)

4. Perform five sets, alternating sides.

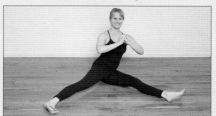

Take your triangle on a walk progression (B)

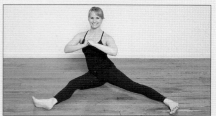

Take your triangle on a walk progression (C)

Upavistha Konasana pancakes

1. Come into a seated straddle position. Hold on to a block and reach your arms overhead.

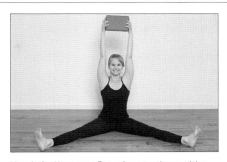

Upavistha Konasana Pancakes starting position

2. Maintain the external rotation of your femurs as you hinge forward with your torso. Try to maintain a neutral spine and keep your arms in line with your ears as you do this.

3. Return to the starting position. Perform five repetitions.

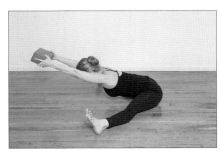

Hinge forward

4. Once you have practiced this exercise moving down the center, you can add rotation. To do this, rotate your chest to the right and hinge forward over your right leg. Return to center and repeat on the left side. Perform five sets, alternating sides.

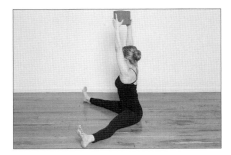

Rotate chest right

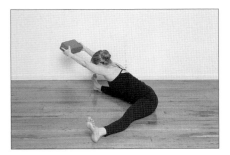

Hinge forward and rotate right

Lower-body emphasis sequence B

Ninety-ninety transitions

1. Come into a tall kneeling position.

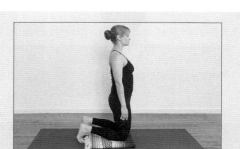

Tall kneeling

Reach your arms out to the sides and make fists with your hands. Try to bring your right heel to your right buttock and hover your right knee, so you are balancing on your left leg.

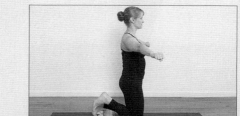

Arms out to sides with fists

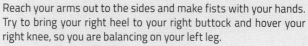

Right heel to right buttock

2. Move your right leg around randomly through space to challenge your balance on your left side.

3. Repeat steps one and two on the second side.

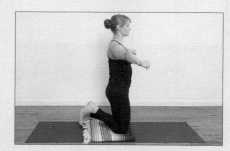

Move your right leg around

4. Come into a tall kneeling position. Reach your arms out to the sides and make fists with your hands. Try to bring your right heel to your right buttock and hover your right knee, so you are balancing on your left leg. Keeping your right leg parallel, bring it forward, so your knee moves towards your chest into hip flexion. Pause for a breath.

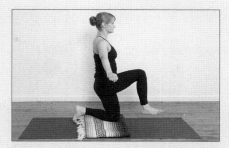

Right knee to chest

Place your right foot on the floor in front of you. Move your right leg through hip flexion and hip extension for up to three rounds, pausing in each position to balance on the left leg.

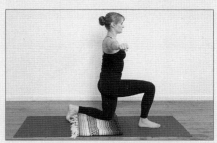

Right foot planted in a half kneeling position

5. Pause in a half-kneeling position with the right leg forward and the left leg back. Tuck the back toes under and hover the back knee an inch off the ground.

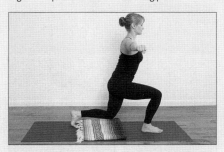

Back knee hovers

6. Come into a standing position and bring your left knee towards your chest. Try not to touch your left foot to the ground as you do this.

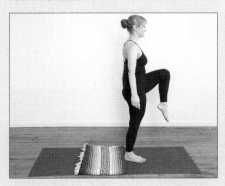

Stand with knee to chest

7. Step your left foot back and lower into a ninety-ninety hover.

8. Repeat steps four through seven on the second side.

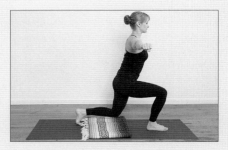

Ninety-ninety hover

Section 3 Upper-body emphasis

Upper-body emphasis sequence A

Wrist loading

1. Come into four-point kneeling with your knees under your hips and your hands under your shoulders. If you experience wrist discomfort, walk your hands slightly forward of your shoulders.

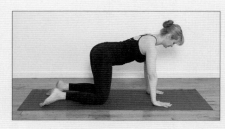

Four-point kneeling

2. Turn your fingers to face outwards with straight elbows. Hold for a count of two.

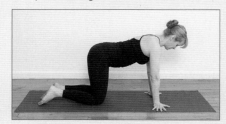

Fingers turned outward

3. Turn your fingers to face inwards with straight elbows. Hold for a count of two.

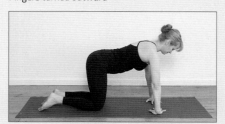

Fingers turned inward

4. Turn your fingers to face backwards towards your knees with straight elbows. Hold for a count of two.

5. Repeat steps two through four for four cycles.

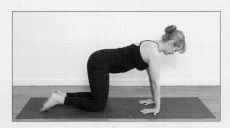

Fingers facing backwards

Wrist push-ups

1. Come into four-point kneeling with your knees under your hips and your hands under your shoulders. If you experience wrist discomfort, walk your hands slightly forward of your shoulders.

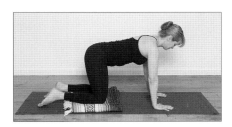

Four-point kneeling

2. With straight elbows, peel the base of your palms and thumbs off the ground. Try to keep your shoulders away from your ears as you perform the exercise.

3. Lower with control. Perform five repetitions.

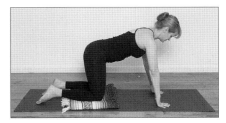

Palms lifted in four-point kneeling

I Dream of Jeannie planks

1. Come into a kneeling forearm plank with your forearms parallel to one another and a block in the second position between your lower legs.

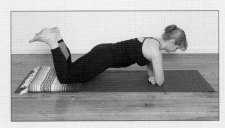

Kneeling forearm plank with block

2. Rotate to the left as you reach your right arm up to the ceiling.

3. Rotate center to return to the starting position.

4. Repeat on the second side. Perform five sets, alternating sides.

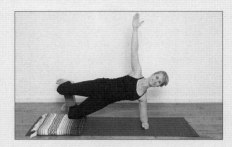

Rotate and reach

Upper-body emphasis sequence B

Quadruped thoracic rotation with prayer hands

1. Come into four-point kneeling with your knees under your hips and your hands under your shoulders.

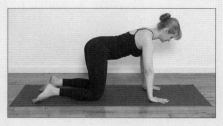

Four-point kneeling

2. Bring your right thumb to your sternum.

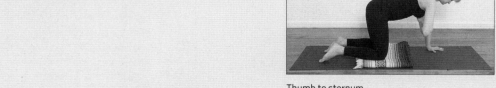

Thumb to sternum

3. Rotate your chest to the right.

4. Return to the starting position.

5. Perform five repetitions and repeat on the second side.

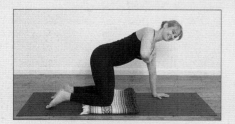

Rotate your chest with thumb to sternum

Quadruped thoracic rotation with shoulder abduction

1. Come into four-point kneeling with your knees under your hips and your hands under your shoulders.

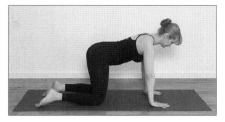

Four-point kneeling

2. Abduct and externally rotate your right shoulder, so your thumb faces the ceiling.

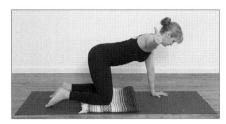

Abduct and externally rotate one shoulder

3. Rotate your chest to the right.

4. Return to the starting position.

5. Perform five repetitions and repeat on the second side.

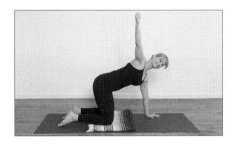

Rotate your chest with shoulder abduction

Quadruped thoracic rotation with block

1. Come into four-point kneeling with your knees under your hips and your hands under your shoulders.

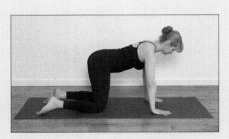

Four-point kneeling

2. Hold on to a cork brick with your right hand. Abduct and externally rotate your right shoulder, so your thumb faces the ceiling.

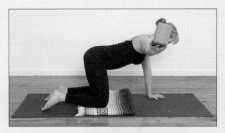

Hold a cork brick and abduct one shoulder

3. Rotate your chest to the right.

4. Return to the starting position.

5. Perform five repetitions and repeat on the second side.

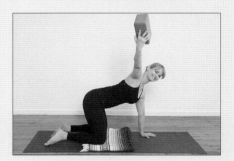

Rotate your chest holding a brick

Sukhasana with horizontal pull aparts

1. Double knot a loop on each end of your stretchy band and sit in a cross-legged position with one hand in each loop.

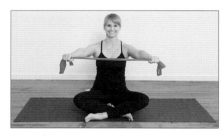

Sit cross legged and hold a band

2. Flex your shoulders to shoulder height. Abduct and retract your shoulders to pull the band apart.

3. Return to the starting position with control.

4. Perform five repetitions.

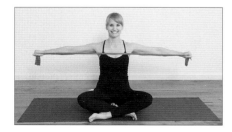

Flex your shoulders to shoulder height

Sukhasana with overhead pull aparts

1. Double knot a loop on each end of your stretchy band and sit in a cross-legged position with one hand in each loop.

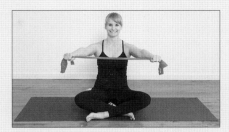

Sit cross legged and hold a band

2. Lift your arms overhead.

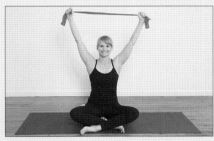

Lift your arms overhead

3. Pull the band apart until your arms are horizontal with the floor.

4. Return to the starting position with control.

5. Perform five repetitions.

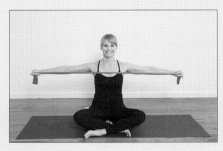

Pull the band apart

Cartwheel arms

1. Double knot a loop on each end of your stretchy band and sit in a cross-legged position with one hand in each loop.

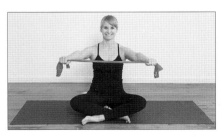

Sit cross legged and hold a band

2. Lift your arms overhead. Laterally flex your spine to the right, so your right hand connects to the floor.

3. Pull against the band to lift your left arm up towards the ceiling. Lower with control. Side bend left so left hand connects to the floor.

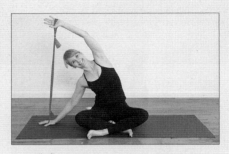

Laterally flex your spine

4. Perform five repetitions. Come to center and repeat on the second side.

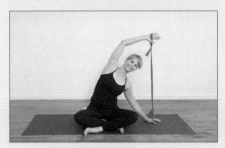

Laterally flex your spine to the second side

Cartwheel arms with rotation

1. Double knot a loop on each end of your stretchy band and sit in a cross-legged position with one hand in each loop.

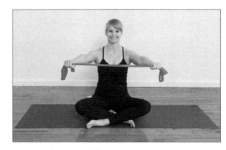

Sit cross legged and hold a band

2. Lift your arms overhead. Laterally flex your spine to the right, so your right hand connects to the floor. Place your left hand behind your head.

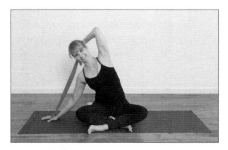

Laterally flex your spine

3. Keeping tension on the band, rotate your chest towards the ceiling.

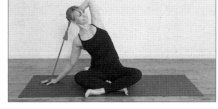

Rotate your chest towards the ceiling

4. Rotate your chest towards the floor. As you do this, the band will go slack.

5. Perform five repetitions. Come to center and repeat on the second side.

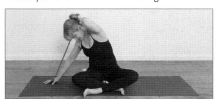

Rotate your chest towards the floor

Cartwheel arms with around the world

1. Double knot a loop on each end of your stretchy band and sit in a cross-legged position with one hand in each loop.

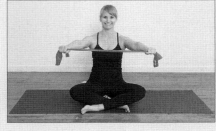

Sit cross legged and hold a band

2. Lift your arms overhead. Laterally flex your spine to the left, so your left hand connects to the floor.

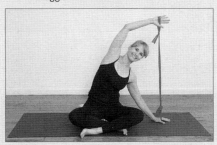

Laterally flex your spine to one side

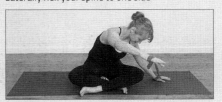

Begin to rotate towards the middle

3. Pass through the middle and place your right hand on the floor, so your spine is in lateral flexion.

4. Come to seated. Perform five repetitions.

5. Reverse directions.

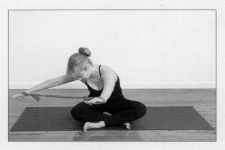

Pass through the middle

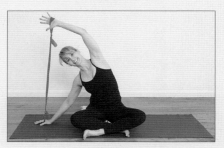

Laterally flex your spine to the second side

Track 5 Preparatory exercises in standing

Section 1 Spine emphasis

Spine emphasis sequence A

Sukhasana to stand transitions

1. Start sitting in a cross-legged position on your mat.

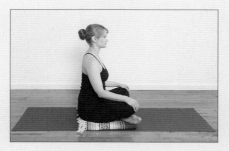

Sit cross legged

2. Rock forward on to your knees.

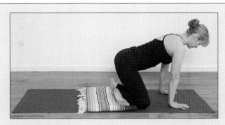

Rock forward

3. Bring your shins parallel to come into four-point kneeling.

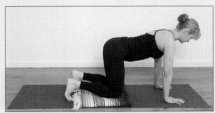

Come into four-point kneeling

4. Tuck your toes under and move your pelvis back towards your heels.

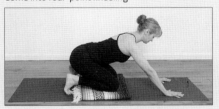

Tuck your toes and move pelvis towards heels

5. Come into tall kneeling with your toes tucked under.

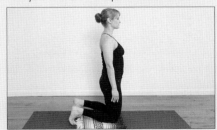

Tall kneeling toes tucked under

6. Keeping your right femur parallel, pull your right heel to your right sit bone.

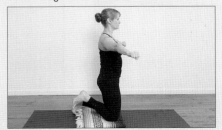

Right heel to right sit bone

7. Bring the right knee towards your chest, so you are balancing on your left leg.

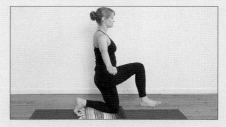

Right knee to chest

8. Lower your right foot to the floor to come into a half-kneeling position.

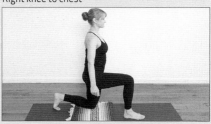

Half-kneeling position

9. Reach your arms out to the sides and make fists with your hands. Try to bring your right heel to your right buttock and hover your right knee, so you are balancing on your left leg. Keeping your right leg parallel, bring it forward, so your knee moves towards your chest into hip flexion. Pause for a breath.

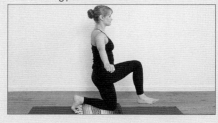

Balance on left leg

10. Place your right foot on the floor in front of you. Move your right leg through hip flexion and hip extension for up to three rounds, pausing in each position to balance on the left leg.

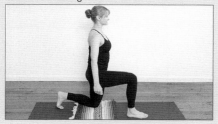

Place right foot on the floor in front of you

11. Press into the ground to hover your left knee an inch off the floor.

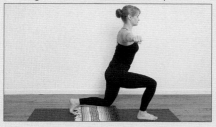

Back knee hovers

12. Stand up by bringing the left foot forward, so it is in line with the right foot.

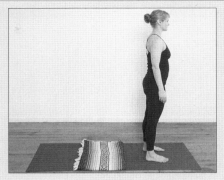

Stand up

13. Reverse the order to come back the way you came, so you end sitting on the mat the same way you started.

14. Repeat on the second side, leading with the left leg. Perform two sets, alternating sides.

Standing hip circles

1. Stand in Tadasana with your core and glutes engaged. Make fists with your hands and create tension as if you were gripping a bar. Feel that tension transfer through your arms, shoulders, and chest.

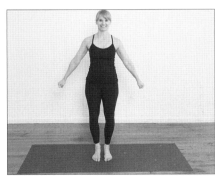

Tadasana with hands in fists

2. Lift your right knee to your chest.

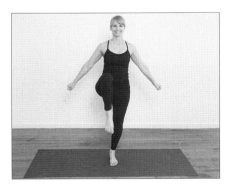

Lift your right knee to your chest

3. Abduct your right hip as you try to keep the rest of your body still.

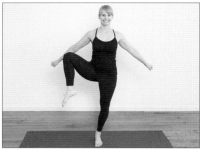

Abduct your right hip

4. Internally rotate your right hip as you try to keep the rest of your body still.

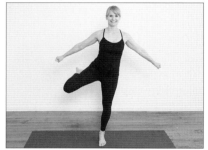

Internally rotate right hip

5. Adduct your right hip as you try to keep the rest of your body still.

6. Return to the starting position with your right hip in flexion.

7. Repeat steps three through six for three to five cycles. Reverse directions.

8. Perform on the left side.

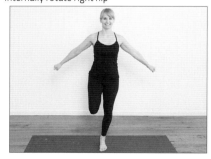

Adduct right hip

Standing roll down

1. Stand in Tadasana.

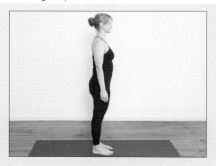

Tadasana

2. Nod your chin forward and allow your spine to move into flexion vertebra by vertebra as your arms reach for the floor. Allow your knees to bend as much as needed to perform this movement. Depending on your mobility, your hands may or may not touch the floor.

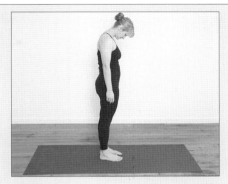

Rolldown (A)

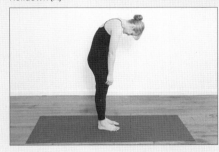

Rolldown (B)

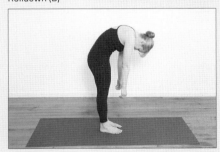

Rolldown (C)

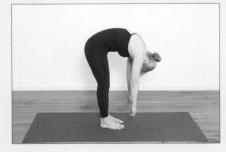

Rolldown (D)

3. Soften your knees at the bottom and roll through your spine to return to the starting position.

4. Perform three to five repetitions.

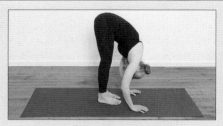

Soften your knees at the bottom

Dripping sideways

1. Stand in Tadasana.

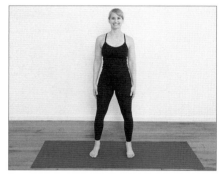

Tadasana

2. Drop your right ear towards your right shoulder.

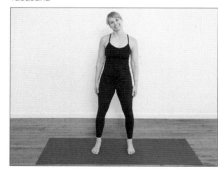

Ear to shoulder

3. Allow your spine to move into lateral flexion vertebra by vertebra.

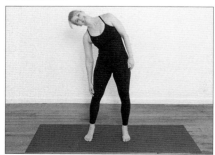

Lateral flexion (A)

4. As your right arm reaches for the floor, your left arm reaches overhead. Allow your knees to bend as much as needed to perform this movement.

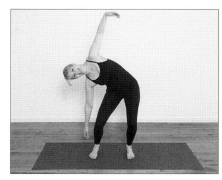

Lateral flexion (B)

5. Depending on your mobility, your right hand may or may not touch the floor.

6. Roll back up the way you came to move out of lateral flexion and return to the starting position.

7. Perform three to five repetitions and repeat on second side.

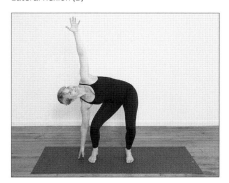

Lateral flexion (C)

Spine emphasis sequence B

Standing rib-cage circles

1. Stand with your feet about four-feet apart. Wrap your arms tightly around your rib cage.

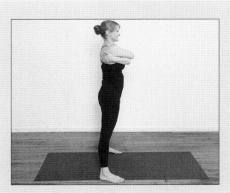

Arms wrapped around rib cage

2. Flex your spine while keeping your hips neutral, because there will be a tendency to hip hinge.

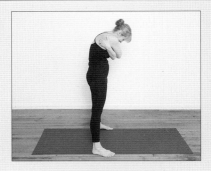

Flex your spine with a neutral pelvis

3. Rotate to the right, while maintaining spinal flexion.

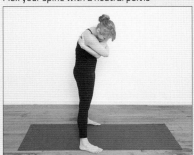

Rotate and flex your spine to the right

4. Laterally flex your spine to the right.

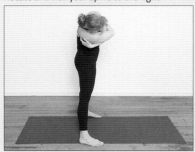

Laterally flex your spine to the right

5. Rotate and extend your spine to the left.

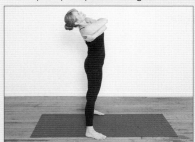

Rotate and extend your spine to the left

6. Extend your thoracic spine.

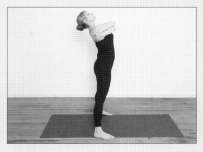

Extend your thoracic spine

7. Rotate and flex your spine to the left.

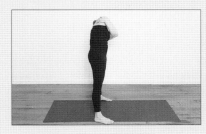

Laterally flex your spine to the left side

8. Transition to spinal flexion, so you are in the position described in step two.

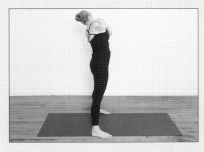

Rotate and flex your spine to the second side

9. Repeat steps two through eight in the opposite direction.

10. Perform three to five rounds, reversing directions each time.

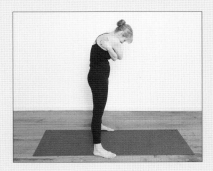

Return to spinal flexion

Zombie bounces

1. Stand in Tadasana.

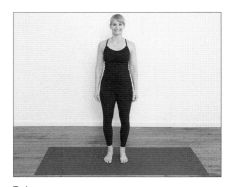

Tadasana

2. Nod your chin forward and allow your spine to move into flexion vertebra by vertebra as your arms reach for the floor. Allow your knees to bend as much as needed to perform this movement. Pause when your hands are at the tops of your kneecaps.

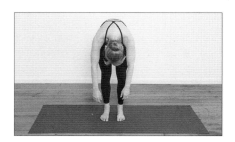

Flex your spine

3. Perform a gentle bouncing movement with your torso. Allow your spine to rotate to the right and left as you do this.

4. Pause in the middle and roll down until your fingertips graze your shins.

5. Perform a gentle bouncing movement with your torso. Allow your spine to rotate to the right and left as you do this.

6. Soften your knees at the bottom and roll through your spine to return to the starting position.

7. Perform three to five repetitions.

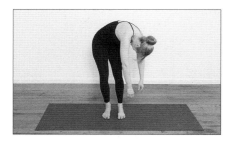

Gently bounce to one side

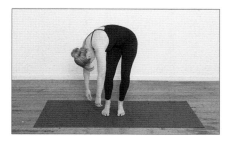

Gently bounce to the second side

Karate Kid Cat Cow

1. Place two blocks two-inches apart. Stand on the blocks, so the balls of your feet are on one brick and your heels are on the second brick and there is a space underneath your arches.

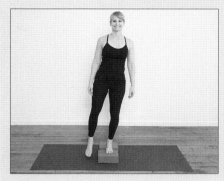

Stand on two blocks

2. Use your hands to bring your right knee to your chest. Notice your range of motion.

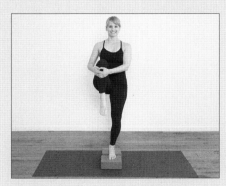

Bring knee to chest

3. Release your hands from your leg and try to maintain the position outlined in step two.

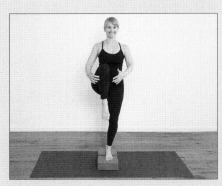

Knee to chest without hands

4. Take your arms out to your sides and internally rotate your shoulders. Sweep your arms forward as you flex your spine.

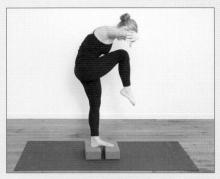

Stand on blocks with spinal flexion

5. Externally rotate your shoulders and sweep your arms back as you pull your right heel to your right buttock.

6. Repeat steps three through five up to three times.

7. Perform on second side.

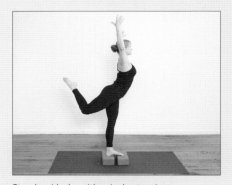

Stand on blocks with spinal extension

Section 2 Lower-body emphasis

Lower-body emphasis sequence A

Cobbler's Pose to stand

1. Stack two blocks on the floor. Come into a seated position on the blocks with the soles of your feet together.

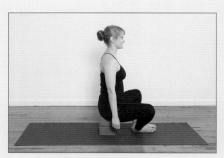

Seated Cobblers Pose

2. Hinge forward and try to hover your pelvis off the blocks.

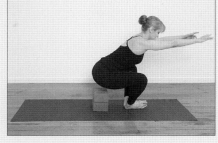

Cobblers Pose hinge forward

3. Once you are comfortable with hovering, try to come into a standing position.

4. Lower with control.

5. Perform three to five reps.

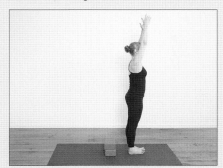

Cobblers Pose standing

Sukhasana Pose to stand

1. Stack two blocks on the floor. Come into a seated position on the blocks with your ankles crossed in Sukhasana.

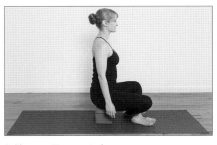

Sukhasana Pose seated

2. Hinge forward and try to hover your pelvis off the blocks.

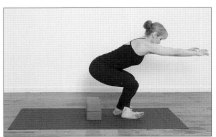

Sukhasana Pose hinge forward

3. Once you are comfortable with hovering, try to come into a standing position.

4. Lower with control.

5. Perform three to five reps.

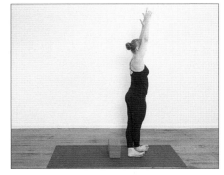

Sukhasana Pose standing

Skandasana slides

1. Stand with your heels together, your toes apart, and your right foot on top of a folded blanket.

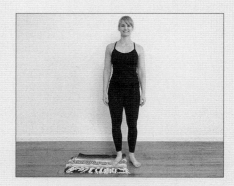

Stand with heels together

2. Bend your left knee and slide your right leg out to the side at a 45-degree angle as you reach your arms forward for balance. The right femur should stay in external rotation. Only go out as far as you can come back.

3. Return to the starting position.

4. Perform three to five repetitions and repeat on the second side.

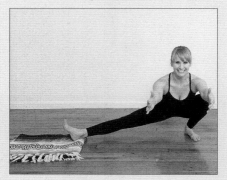

Slide one leg to the side

Lower-body emphasis sequence B

Sun salute with blanket slide

1. Stand in Tadasana with your right foot on a blanket and two blocks in front of you at third setting.

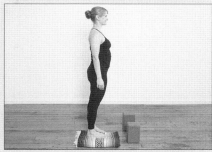

Tadasana with foot on blanket

2. Sweep your arms out to the sides and up towards the ceiling as you look up at your hands.

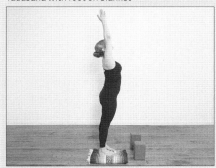

Reach arms to ceiling

3. Sweep your arms down by your sides as you reach your hands forward to touch the blocks.

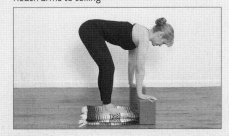

Forward Fold

4. Bend your knees and lift your chest.

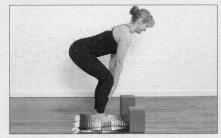

Knees bent with chest lifted

5. Return to Forward Fold.

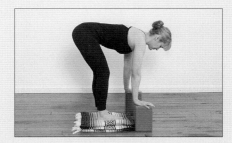

Forward Fold

6. Bend your left knee and slide your right foot back into Crescent Lunge.

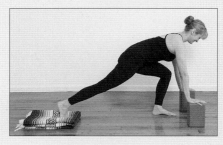

Crescent Lunge with blanket

7. Pause in Crescent Lunge and lift your arms up towards the ceiling.

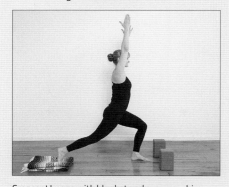

Crescent Lunge with blanket and arms reaching

8. Bring your hands back down to the bricks as you slide your right leg forward into the bottom of a pistol squat.

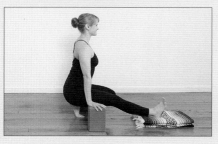

Pistol squat with blanket

9. Push your hands into the bricks and slide your right leg back to return to Forward Fold.

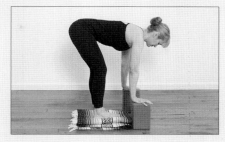

Forward Fold

10. Repeat steps one through nine on the second side with the blanket under your left foot.

Section 3 Upper-body emphasis

Upper-body emphasis sequence A

Elbows forward, hands back

1. Stand in Tadasana. Bring a strap behind your head and hold on to it with your arms in a cactus position.

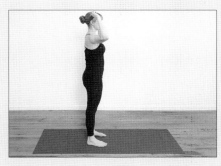

Tadasana with strap behind head

2. Pull your elbows forward, so your elbows are in your peripheral vision.

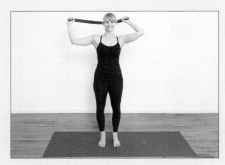

Elbows pulled forward (A)

3. Try to keep your body still as you pull the strap side to side.

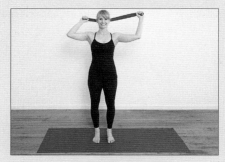

Elbows pulled forward (B)

4. Perform 8 to 10 rounds.

Halo circles

1. Stand in Tadasana. Bring a strap behind your head and hold on to it with your arms in a cactus position. Pull your elbows forward, so your elbows are in your peripheral vision.

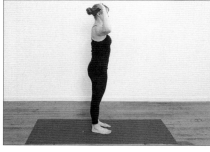

Tadasana with strap behind head

2. Pull on the strap to take your hands to the right.

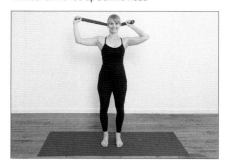

Strap to the right

3. Pull on the strap to take your hands up overhead.

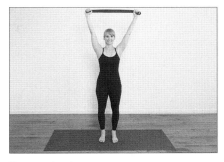

Strap overhead

4. Pull on the strap to take your hands to the left.

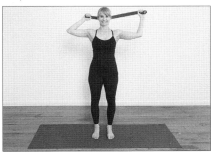

Strap to the left

5. Pull on the strap to take your hands back down in a circular motion to the starting position. Try to keep your body still as you do this.

6. Perform 8 to 10 repetitions and reverse direction.

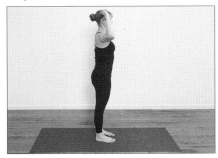

Return strap to starting position.

Bottom circles

1. Stand in Tadasana. Bring a strap behind your thighs and hold on to it with the shoulders in internal rotation.

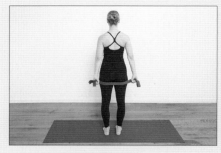

Tadasana with strap behind thighs

2. Pull on the strap to take your hands to the right and bend your elbows.

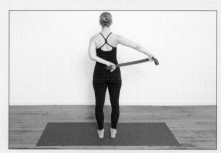

Pull strap to the right

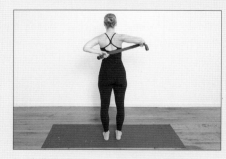

Bend elbows

3. Pull on the strap to take your hands to the left and straighten your elbows. Try to keep your body still as you do this.

4. Perform 8 to 10 repetitions and reverse directions.

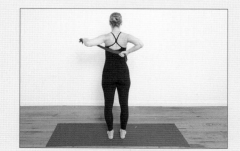

Pull strap to the left

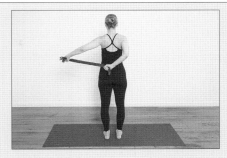

Straighten elbows

Serving master tea

1. Stand in Tadasana, holding a block in your right hand. Bend your right elbow and extend your wrist, so the block is balancing on the palm of your right hand.

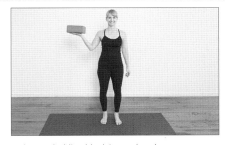

Tadasana holding block in one hand

2. Press the block overhead while maintaining wrist extension and shoulder external rotation.

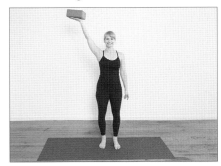

Block overhead

3. Internally rotate your shoulder while in the overhead position.

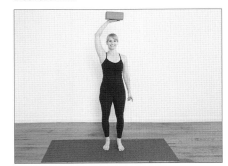

Internally rotate shoulder with block overhead

4. Laterally flex your spine to the left as you lower your right arm while keeping the block balanced on your palm.

5. Return to the starting position.

6. Perform three to five repetitions and repeat on the second side.

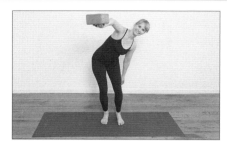

Laterally flex spine and lower arm (A)

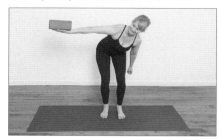

Laterally flex spine and lower arm (B)

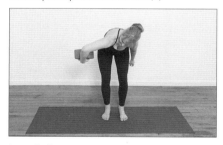

Laterally flex spine and lower arm (C)

Upper-body emphasis sequence B

Talk to the hands

1. Stand in Tadasana with your elbows bent at 90 degrees and a block between your forearms in the second position and a strap looped around your hands. Your forearms should be supinated.

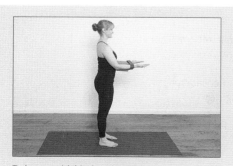

Tadasana with block and strap

2. Flex your shoulders while maintaining forearm supination and keeping your torso still.

3. Lower your arms to return to the starting position. Perform 8 to 10 repetitions.

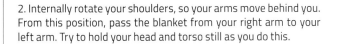

Shoulder flexion with block and strap

Yoga sommelier

1. Stand in Tadasana with a block between your thighs and a blanket draped over your right forearm. Bend your elbows to 90 degrees with the blanket draped over your right arm, your shoulders in maximal external rotation, and your forearms in supination.

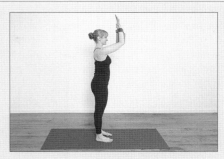

Tadasana with blanket draped over arm

2. Internally rotate your shoulders, so your arms move behind you. From this position, pass the blanket from your right arm to your left arm. Try to hold your head and torso still as you do this.

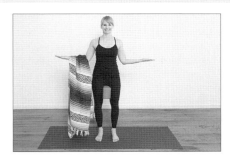

Pass blanket behind you

3. Return to the starting position with the blanket draped over your left arm, your shoulders in external rotation, and your forearms in supination.

4. Repeat steps two and three to pass the blanket back to your right arm.

5. Perform 8 to 10 rounds, alternating sides each time.

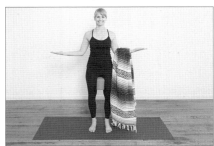

Tadasana with blanket draped over other arm

Active shoulder extension sequence

1. Perform a check of active shoulder extension by standing in Tadasana with a block between your thighs. Hold your head and torso still as you internally rotate, retract, and maximally extend your shoulders with your elbows straight. Notice your range of motion in this position. Lower your arms.

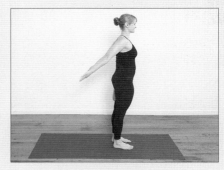

Active shoulder extension check

2. Hold on to a strap behind your thighs. Keep your head and torso still as you pull the strap apart and internally rotate, retract, and maximally extend your shoulders with your elbows straight. Continue to tug on the strap and keep your body still as you hold this position for up to 10 focused breaths.

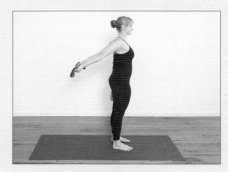

Active shoulder extension with strap

3. Hold on to a block between your hands. Keep your head and torso still as you tug on the block and internally rotate, retract, and maximally extend your shoulders with your elbows straight. Continue to pull the block apart and keep your body still as you hold this position for up to 10 focused breaths.

4. Perform a recheck by repeating the movements outlined in step one. Notice if your active open chain range of motion has increased.

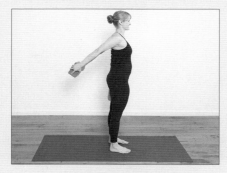

Active shoulder extension with block

Track 6 Pose sequence

Section 1 Spine emphasis

Flowing Gate Pose sequence

Gate Pose (Parighasana)

1. Come to tall kneeling in the middle of your mat with one block to each side of the mat.

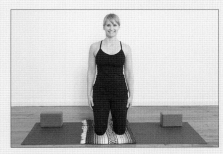

Tall kneeling

2. Take your left leg out to the side. Place your left hand on your hip and reach your right arm up to the ceiling.

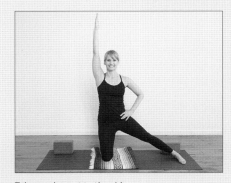

Take one leg out to the side

3. Laterally flex your spine to the left.

4. Laterally flex your spine to the right, so your right hand touches the block and your left arm reaches overhead.

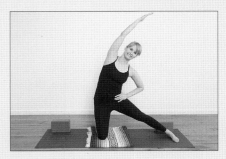

Laterally flex to one side

Gate Pose pass the brick

1. Pick up the block with your right hand.

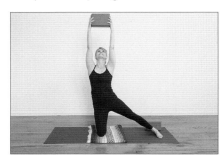

Pick up block with your right hand

2. Reach it overhead to pass off to your left hand. Allow your gaze to follow the brick.

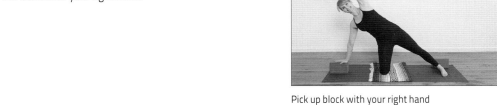

Pass block overhead

3. Place the block on the floor behind your left leg and laterally flex your spine to the left as your right arm reaches overhead.

4. Repeat this process three to five times.

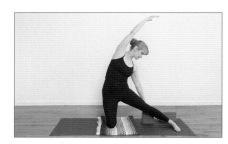

Place block on side

Floating Gate Pose

1. Pause with your right hand on the block, your left arm reaching alongside your left ear and your left leg extended out to the side.

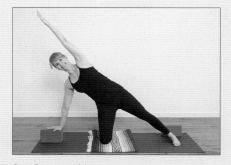

Gate Pose transition

2. Abduct your left hip, so your foot lifts off the floor. Reach your left arm up to the ceiling.

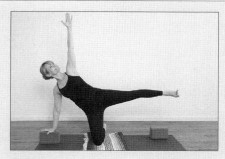

Abduct one hip

3. Tuck your right toes under and hover your right hand an inch off the block.

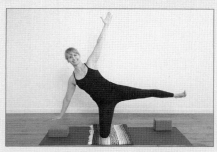

Hover hand with hip abducted

4. Place your right hand back on the block and lower your left foot to the floor.

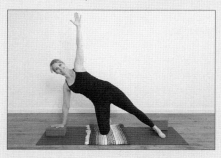

Place hand on block and foot on floor

5. Laterally flex your spine to the left and place your left hand on your left hip.

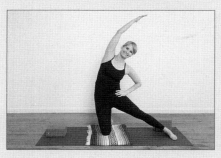

Laterally flex your spine

Gate Pose with thoracic rotation

1. Place your right hand at the back of your head.

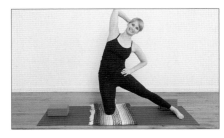

Hand behind head

2. Rotate your spine to the right, so your chest is angled towards the ceiling.

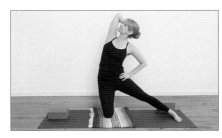

Rotate and extend your spine

3. Rotate and flex your spine to the left, so your chest is angled towards the floor.

4. Repeat this process three to five times.

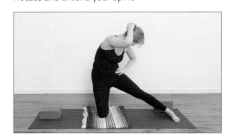

Rotate and flex your spine

Single knee balance to tall kneeling

1. Come up to center and reach your arms out to the sides. Make fists with your hands.

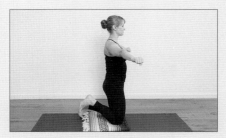

Hover left foot off ground

How to design a Yoga Deconstructed® class

2. Hover your left foot off the ground and move it around, so you are balancing over your right leg. Return to tall kneeling and repeat the entire sequence on the second side.

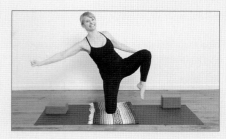

Hover left foot off ground

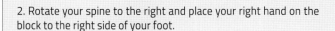

Flowing Camel Pose sequence

Camel Pose with thoracic rotation

1. Come to tall kneeling with your toes tucked under in the middle of your mat with two blocks on the third setting to the outside of each foot and in line with your heels.

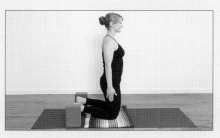

Tall kneeling toes tucked under

2. Rotate your spine to the right and place your right hand on the block to the right side of your foot.

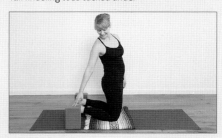

Rotate and place hand on block

3. Return to center and repeat step two on the left. Perform up to five rounds, alternating sides each time.

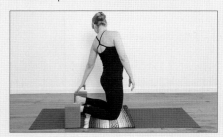

Rotate and place hand on block second side

211

Camel Pose with arm reaches

1. Come to tall kneeling with your toes tucked under in the middle of your mat with two blocks on the third setting in line with the outer edge of your heels.

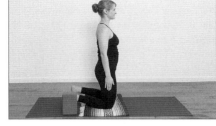

Tall kneeling toes tucked under

2. Rotate your spine to the right and place your right hand on the block to the right side of your foot as you reach your left arm overhead.

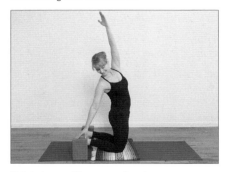

Rotate to one side arm overhead

3. Return to center and repeat step one on the left. Perform up to five rounds, alternating sides each time.

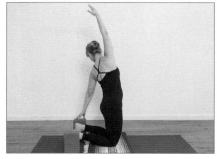

Rotate to second side arm overhead

Camel Pose around the world

1. Come to tall kneeling with your toes tucked under in the middle of your mat with two blocks on the third setting in line with the outer edge of your heels.

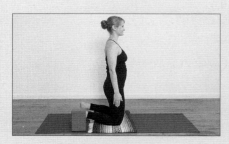

Tall kneeling toes tucked under

2. Rotate your spine to the right and place your right hand on the block to the right side of your foot as you reach your left arm overhead.

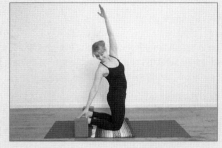

Rotate and place hand on block with arm reaching overhead

3. Reach your right arm up by your right ear as you rotate left, so your spine is in thoracic extension with your chest angled towards the ceiling.

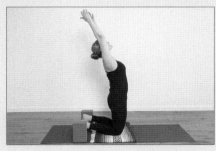

Thoracic extension to middle

4. Rotate left, so your left hand touches the brick near your left heel and your right arm reaches overhead.

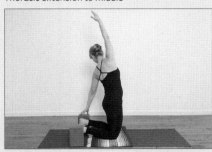

Rotate and place hand on block with arm reaching overhead second side

5. Reach your left arm up by your left ear as you rotate right, so your spine is in thoracic extension with your chest angled towards the ceiling.

6. Repeat steps one through four for three rounds.

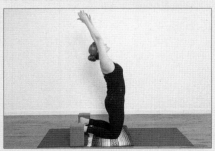

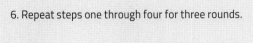
Thoracic extension to middle

Camel Pose pass the block

1. Come to tall kneeling with your toes tucked under in the middle of your mat with one block on the third setting in line with the outer edge of your right heel.

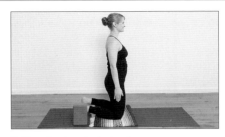

Tall kneeling toes tucked under

2. Rotate your spine to the right and place your right hand on the block as your left arm reaches overhead.

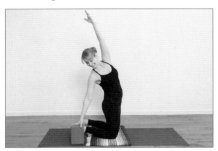

Rotate and place hand on block with arm reaching overhead

3. Pick up the block with your right hand as you move into thoracic extension.

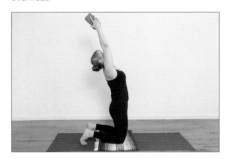

Thoracic extension to middle with block

4. Pass the block to your left hand as you laterally flex your spine to the left to place the brick on the ground to the left side of your body.

5. Repeat steps one through four for three rounds.

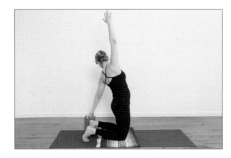

Rotate and place hand on block with arm reaching overhead second side

Static Camel Pose with pull up

1. Come to tall kneeling with your toes tucked under in the middle of your mat.

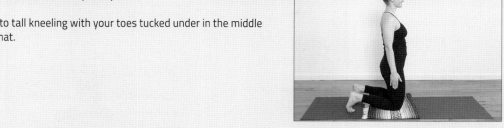

Tall kneeling toes tucked under

2. Reach your arms up towards the ceiling like you're grabbing a pull-up bar.

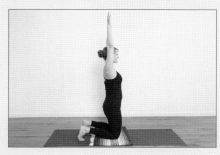

Tall kneeling arms reaching overhead

3. Engage your glutes and abdominals, and create fists with your hands as you bend your elbows, slide your shoulders down your back, and extend your thoracic spine to create global tension. Perform three repetitions.

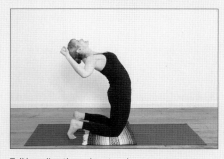

Tall kneeling thoracic extension

4. Pause in thoracic extension and lightly touch your heels with your hands. Hold this position for three to five breaths.

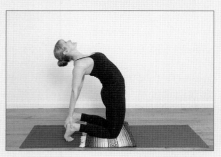

Full Camel Pose

Floating Half Moon sequence

Warrior II to Extended Side Angle Pose to Half Moon

1. Come into Warrior II with your left knee bent with a block near your left foot.

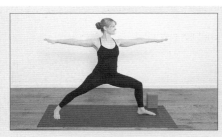

Warrior II

2. Place your left forearm on your left thigh and reach your right arm by your ear to come into Extended Side Angle Pose.

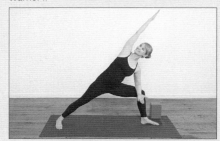

Extended Side Angle Pose

3. Shift your weight onto your left foot and lift your right foot off the floor to come into Half Moon.

4. Transition from Half Moon to Extended Side Angle Pose to Warrior II and repeat on the other side.

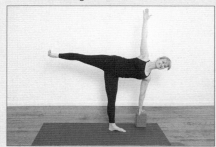

Half Moon Pose

Jedi warrior squat to Half Moon

1. Take your feet out slightly wider than hip-width apart with your right toes pointing at a 45-degree angle and your left toes pointing slightly inwards. Clasp your hands together and bend your knees to lower into a squat stance.

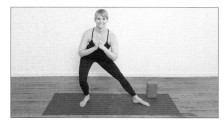

Squat stance with one foot turned in and one foot turned out

2. Shift your weight into your left foot and allow your right knee to straighten as needed.

3A. Shift your weight into your right foot, so your right knee bends and your left knee straightens as needed.

3B. Shift your weight back into your left foot.

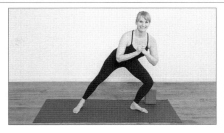

Weight shift into front foot

4. Keep your weight over your left foot and straighten both knees to come into a floating Half Moon with your arms reaching out by your sides.

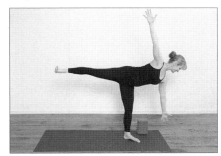

Floating Half Moon Pose

5. Bend your left knee to place your right foot on the ground, clasp your hands, and bend your knees and shift your weight into your right leg.

6. Repeat steps two through five for three rounds and perform on second side.

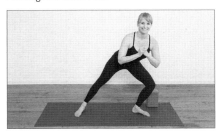

Weight shift hands clasped

Sideways Gorilla hops

1. Stand with your feet slightly wider than hip-width apart. Bend your knees and send your hips back.

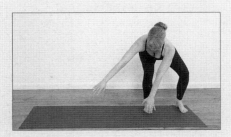

Knees bent with hips back

2. Place your left hand and then your right hand on the ground, one hand at a time.

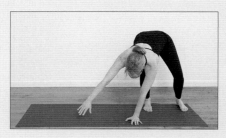

Hands to floor

3. Push through your left foot and then your right foot to hop your feet to the right, so your weight shifts over your hands.

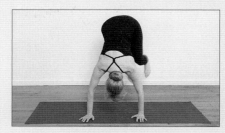

Initial foot push off

4. Float your feet to the ground with control. Repeat steps one through three for three to five rounds and then reverse directions, so you end in the starting position.

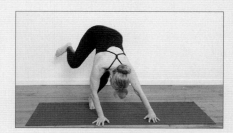

Land your feet

Standing Apanasana to Warrior III sequence

1. Stand in Tadasana.

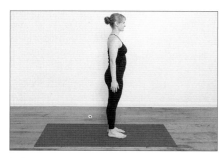

Tadasana

2. Pull your right knee to your chest.

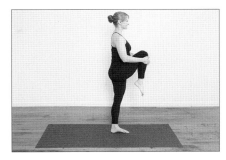

Pull knee to chest

3. Release your leg and try to keep your right knee at your chest.

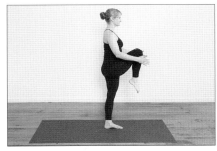

Knee to chest without hands

4. Dorsiflex your right ankle and extend your right knee while maintaining hip flexion in your right leg.

5. Reach your arms up towards the ceiling and bring your right knee to your chest (no photo).

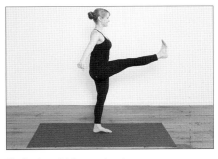

Hip flexion with knee extension

6. Keep your right heel close to your right buttock as you hinge at your hips and lower your torso towards the floor.

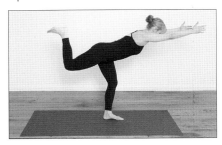

Hip extension with knee flexion

7. Extend and bend your right knee three times.

8. Pause with your right knee extended and step back into Crescent Lunge.

9. Shift your weight forward to return to the position outlined in step three. Try not to let your right foot touch the floor as you do this.

10. Repeat steps one through nine on the second side.

11. Perform two to three rounds, alternating sides each time.

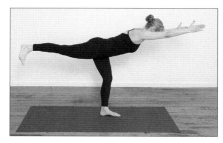

Hip extension with knee extension

Section 3 Upper-body emphasis

Wide-legged Side Plank into Wild Thing sequence

Wide-legged Plank with ankle rotation

1. Come into a plank position with your wrists under your shoulders and your feet hip-width apart.

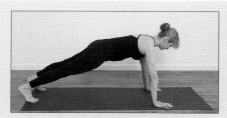

Plank Pose

2. Lower your head, so you can see your feet.

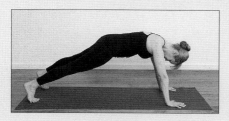

Plank Pose with head lowered

3. Maintain ankle dorsiflexion as you shift your weight to the outer edge of your right foot and the inner edge of your left foot.

4. Return to center and repeat on the second side.

5. Perform five rounds, alternating sides each time.

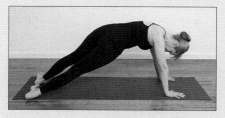

Plank Pose with head lowered and weight shift of feet

Alternating Wide-legged Side Plank

1. Come into a plank position with your wrists under your shoulders and your feet hip-width apart.

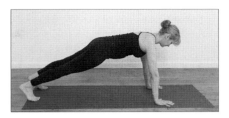

Plank Pose

2. Maintain ankle dorsiflexion as you shift your weight to the outer edge of your right foot and the inner edge of your left foot.

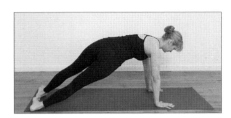

Plank Pose with weight shift of feet

3. Pause in this position and reach your left arm up to the ceiling to assume a side plank.

4. Lower your left hand to the floor and shift your weight back to center.

5. Repeat on second side. Perform five rounds, alternating sides each time.

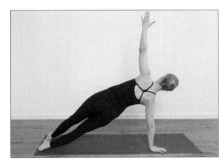

Side Plank

Alternating Wide-legged Side Plank into Kickstand or Wild Thing

1. Come into a plank position with your wrists under your shoulders and your feet hip-width apart.

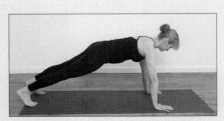

Plank Pose

2. Maintain ankle dorsiflexion as you shift your weight to the outer edge of your left foot and the inner edge of your right foot.

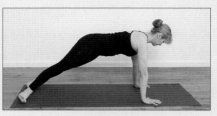

Plank Pose with weight shift of feet

3. Pause in this position and reach your right arm up to the ceiling to assume a side plank.

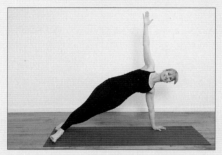

Side Plank

4. Bend your right knee and lift it up towards the right side of your chest.

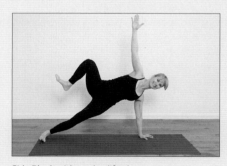

Side Plank with top leg lifted

5. Place your right foot on the floor in plantar flexion behind your left leg.

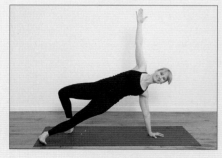

Side Plank with top leg planted behind anchoring leg

6. If it feels available to you, extend your spine and hips to move into Wild Thing.

7. To come out of Wild Thing, flex your hips and pivot to center to return to a wide-legged plank.

8. Repeat steps two through seven on the other side.

9. Perform three rounds, alternating sides each time.

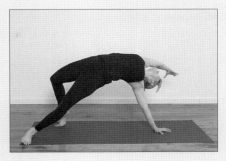

Wild Thing

Purvottanasana Sequence

Purvottanasana with Cat Cow

1. Come into a seated position with knees bent, feet flat on the floor, and forearms resting on two blocks on the second setting. If available, place a third block or ball between your knees.

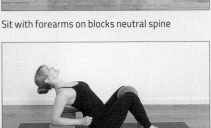

Sit with forearms on blocks neutral spine

2. Push your forearms into the blocks and extend your thoracic spine.

Sit with forearms on blocks spinal extension

3. Lower your head and flex your spine.

4. Perform three to five rounds.

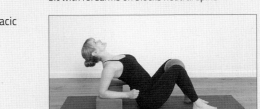

Sit with forearms on blocks spinal flexion

Purvottanasana on forearms

1. Come into a seated position with knees bent, feet flat on the floor, and forearms resting on two blocks in the second setting. If available, place a third block or ball between your knees.

2. Push your forearms into the blocks and retract and depress your shoulder blades.

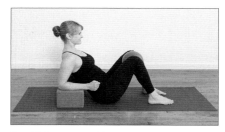

Sit with forearms on blocks neutral spine

3. Press your feet into the floor, posteriorly tilt your pelvis, and lift your hips towards the ceiling.

4. Lower with control. Perform three to five repetitions.

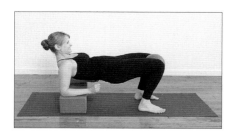

Forearms on blocks hips lifted

Purvottanasana on hands with single leg lift

1. Come into a seated position with knees bent, feet flat on the floor, and hands on the ground. If available, place a block or ball between your knees.

2. Push into your hands and retract and depress your shoulder blades.

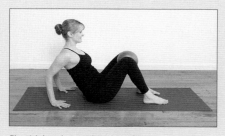

Sit with hands to either side of torso

3. Press your feet into the floor, posteriorly tilt your pelvis, and lift your hips towards the ceiling.

4. Try to maintain a level pelvis as you extend your right knee.

5. Replace your right foot and repeat on the left side.

6. Lower with control. Perform three to five rounds.

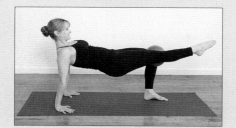

Hips lifted with one knee extended

Finally, I often like to end my classes with Savasana or Legs Up the Wall Pose.

REFERENCES

American College of Physicians, 2017. American College of Physicians issues guideline for treating nonradicular low back pain. Available at: https://www.acponline.org/acp-newsroom/american-college-of-physicians-issues-guideline-for-treating-nonradicular-low-back-pain [Accessed 20 January 2020].

Bharat K, Lenert P, 2017. Joint hypermobility syndrome: recognizing a commonly overlooked cause of chronic pain. *The American Journal of Medicine* 130(6): 640–7.

Celenay ST, Kaya DO, 2017. Effects of spinal stabilization exercises in women with benign joint hypermobility syndrome: a randomized controlled trial. *Rheumatology International* 37: 1461–8.

Centers for Disease Control and Prevention, 2019. Opioids in the Workplace. Available at: https://www.cdc.gov/niosh/topics/opioids/data.html [Accessed 20 January 2020].

Courtney C, et al., 2019. Hypoesthesia after anterior cruciate ligament reconstruction: the relationship between proprioception and vibration perception deficits in individuals greater than one year post-surgery. *The Knee* 26(1): 194–200.

Critchley HD, Garfinkel SN, 2017. Interoception and emotion. *Current Opinion in Psychology* 17:7–14.

Damasio A, et al., 2013. Persistence of feelings and sentience after bilateral damage of the insula. *Cerebral Cortex* 23(4): 833–46.

Davis CM, 2019. Interviewed by Nikki Naab-Levy and Trina Altman, 1 February 2019.

Dubin AE, Patapoutian A, 2010. Nociceptors: the sensors of the pain pathway. *The Journal of Clinical Investigation* 120(11):3760–72.

Eggart M, et al., 2019. Major depressive disorder is associated with impaired interoceptive accuracy: a systematic review. *Brain Sciences* 9(6):131.

Elphinston J, 2019. Interviewed by Nikki Naab-Levy and Trina Altman, 6 August 2019.

Feldenkrais Guild of North America, 2019. About Moshe Feldenkrais. Available at: https://feldenkrais.com/about-moshe-feldenkrais/ [Accessed 20 January 2020].

Gibson J, 2019. Mindfulness, interoception, and the body: a contemporary perspective. *Frontiers in Psychology* [online] https://doi.org/10.3389/fpsyg.2019.02012.

Halperin I, et al., 2014. Roller massager improves range of motion of plantar flexor muscles without subsequent decreases in force parameters. *The International Journal of Sports Physical Therapy* 9(1): 92–102.

Han J, et al., 2016. Assessing proprioception: a critical review of methods. *Journal of Sport and Health Science* 5(1): 80–90.

Hargrove T, 2019. Interviewed by Nikki Naab-Levy and Trina Altman, 7 June 2019.

Hodges PW and Smeets RJ, 2015. Interaction between pain, movement, and physical activity: short-term benefits, long-term consequences, and targets for treatment. *The Clinical Journal of Pain* 31(2): 97–107.

Iyengar BKS, 1979. *Light on yoga: yoga dipika*. New York: Schocken; p. 21.

Jenkinson PM, et al., 2018. Self-reported interoceptive deficits in eating disorders: a meta-analysis of studies using the eating disorder inventory. *Journal of Psychosomatic Research* 110: 38–45.

Keller K and Engelhardt M, 2013. Strength and muscle mass loss with aging process. Age and strength loss. *Muscle, Ligaments and Tendons Journal* 3(4): 346–50.

Kirk JA, et al., 1967. The hypermobility syndrome. Musculoskeletal complaints associated with generalized joint hypermobility. *Annals of Rheumatic Diseases* 26(5): 419–25.

Lehman G, 2018. *Recovery strategies: pain guidebook*; pp. 11–16. Available at: http://www.greglehman.ca/pain-science-workbooks/ [Accessed 20 June 2020].

Lewis JS and Schweinhardt P, 2012. Perceptions of the painful body: the relationship between body perception disturbance, pain and tactile discrimination in complex regional pain syndrome. *European Journal of Pain* 16: 1320–30.

Li JX, et al., 2008. Effects of 16-week Tai Chi intervention on postural stability and proprioception of knee and ankle in older people. *Age and Ageing* 37(5): 575–8.

Lipnicki DM and Byrne DG, 2008. An effect of posture on anticipatory anxiety. *International Journal of Neuroscience* 118(2): 227–37.

Mandelbaum BR, et al., 2005. Effectiveness of a neuromuscular and proprioceptive training program in preventing anterior cruciate ligament injuries in female athletes: 2-year follow-up. *American Journal of Sports Medicine* 33(7): 1003–10.

Martinez-Amat A, et al., 2013. Effects of 12-week proprioception training program on postural stability, gait, and balance in older adults: a controlled clinical trial. *The Journal of Strength & Conditioning Research* 27(8): 2180–8.

Minasny B, 2009. Understanding the process of fascial unwinding. *International Journal of Therapeutic Massage & Bodywork* 2(3): 10–17.

Moseley L, 2016. *Explainer – what is pain?* Available at: https://relief.news/what-is-pain/ [Accessed 20 June 2020].

Nahin RL, 2015. Estimates of pain prevalence and severity in adults: United States, 2012. *Journal of Pain* 16(8): 769–80.

National Institute of Neurological Disorders and Stroke, 2014. Low back pain fact sheet. Available at: https://www.ninds.nih.gov/disorders/patient-caregiver-education/fact-sheets/low-back-pain-fact-sheet [Accessed 20 January 2020].

Phillips K and Clauw DJ, 2011. Central pain mechanisms in chronic pain states – maybe it is all in their head. *Best Practice & Research: Clinical Rheumatology* 25(2): 141–54.

Price CJ, et al., 2019. Immediate effects of interoceptive awareness training through

Mindful Awareness in Body-oriented Therapy (MABT) for women in substance use disorder treatment. *Substance Abuse* 40(1): 102–15.

Prosko S, 2019. Interviewed by Nikki Naab-Levy and Trina Altman, 26 July 2019.

Scheper MC, et al., 2015. Chronic pain in hypermobility syndrome and Ehlers–Danlos syndrome (hypermobility type): it is a challenge. *Journal of Pain Research* 8: 591–601.

Schleip R, 2019. Interviewed by Nikki Naab-Levy and Trina Altman, 8 March 2019.

Schoenfeld B and Contreras B, 2016. Attentional focus for maximizing muscle development. *Strength and Conditioning Journal* 38(1): 27–9.

Sinaki M and Lynn S, 2002. Reducing the risk of falls through proprioceptive dynamic posture training in osteoporotic women with kyphotic posturing: a

randomized pilot study. *American Journal of Physical Medicine & Rehabilitation* 81(4): 241–6.

Sinaki M, et al., 2005. Significant reduction in risk of falls and back pain in osteoporotic-kyphotic women through a spinal proprioceptive extension exercise dynamic (SPEED) program. *Mayo Clinic Proceedings* 80(7): 849–55.

Strauss T., et al., 2019. Touch aversion in patients with interpersonal traumatization. *Depression and Anxiety* 36(7): 635–46.

Suetterlin KJ and Sayer AA, 2014. Proprioception: where are we now? A commentary on clinical assessment, changes across the life course, functional implications and future interventions. *Age and Ageing* 43(3): 313-8.

Swain T and McGwin G, 2016. Yoga-related injuries in the United States

from 2001 to 2014. *Orthopaedic Journal of Sports Medicine* 4(11). doi: 10.1177/2325967116671703.

Wulf G, 2013. Attentional focus and motor learning: a review of 15 years. *International Review of Sport and Exercise Psychology* 6(1): 77–104.

Yoga Alliance, 2016. Highlights from the 2016 Yoga in America Study. Available at: https://www.yogaalliance.org/Learn/About_Yoga/2016_Yoga_in_America_Study/Highlights [Accessed 20 January 2020].

Yoga Journal, 2016. 2016 Yoga in America Study conducted by Yoga Journal and Yoga Alliance. Available at: https://www.yogajournal.com/page/yogainamericastudy [Accessed 20 June 2020].

Zwass-Rupel R, 2019. Interviewed by Nikki Naab-Levy 1 March 2019.

INDEX